AF899887

OXFORD MEDICAL PUBLICATIONS

Alcohol Problems

2

PRACTICAL GUIDES FOR GENERAL PRACTICE

1. *Cervical screening: a practical guide*
   Ann McPherson
2. *A basic formulary for general practice*
   G. B. Grant, D. A. Gregory, and T. D. van Zwanenberg
3. *Radiology*
   Robert F. Bury
4. *Stroke*
   Derick T. Wade
5. *Alcohol problems*
   Peter Anderson, Paul Wallace, and Heather Jones
6. *Breast cancer screening*
   Joan Austoker and John Humphreys
7. *Computers*
   A. W. Willis and T. I. Stewart
8. *Immunizing children*
   Sue Sefi and J. A. Macfarlane

Forthcoming

Non-insulin-dependent diabetes
Ann-Louise Kinmonth

AIDS
John Gallwey and Ann McPherson

Screening tests used in child health surveillance
J. A. Macfarlane and Sue Sefi

Hypertension
T. Schofield

Alcohol Problems

Practical Guides for General Practice 5

PETER ANDERSON
Department of Community Medicine, Oxford
PAUL WALLACE
Department of General Practice,
St Mary's Hospital Medical School, London
HEATHER JONES
Centre for Prevention in Primary Care,
Radcliffe Infirmary, Oxford

Oxford New York Tokyo
OXFORD UNIVERSITY PRESS
1988

Oxford University Press, Walton Street, Oxford OX2 6DP
Oxford New York Toronto
Delhi Bombay Calcutta Madras Karachi
Petaling Jaya Singapore Hong Kong Tokyo
Nairobi Dar es Salaam Cape Town
Melbourne Auckland
and associated companies in
Berlin Ibadan

Oxford is a trade mark of Oxford University Press

Published in the United States
by Oxford University Press, New York

British Library Cataloguing in Publication Data
Anderson, Peter
Alcohol problems.
1. Alcoholic drinks. Consumption. Health aspects
I. Title II. Wallace, Paul III. Jones, Heather IV. Series
613.8'1
ISBN 0–19–261752–4

Library of Congress Cataloging in Publication Data
Anderson, Peter. 1954–
Alcohol problems/Peter Anderson, Paul Wallace, Heather Jones.
— (Practical guides for general practice; 5)
(Oxford medical publications)
Bibliography: (Includes index.)
1. Alcholism—Prevention. 2. Alcholism—Pathophysiology.
3. Drinking of alchololic beverages—Psychological aspects.
I. Wallace, Paul, 1952–. II. Jones, Heather, 1940–.
III. Title. IV. Series. V. Series: Oxford medical publications.
RC565.A515 1988 616.86'1—dc19 88–22632
ISBN 0–19–261752–4 (pbk.):

Set by Computerised Typesetting Services, Redhill, Surrey
Printed in Great Britain
at the University Printing House, Oxford
by David Stanford
Printer to the University

Preface

This book has been written to provide practical guidelines on the management of alcohol problems in general practice. It covers both how to ascertain a patient's alcohol consumption and how to give advice to heavy drinkers to cut down on their drinking.

Alcohol consumption in this country has approximately doubled over the last 20 years. With the increase in the consumption there has been an increase in the many forms of harms—physical, psychological, and social—due to alcohol consumption. Excess alcohol consumption is associated with 30 000 deaths a year and costs this country over £2 billion a year in terms of accidents, lost production at work, and the cost of treating people with alcohol problems.

It has become increasingly clear that in general practice we have an active role to play in the prevention and management of alcohol problems. Indeed, there has been a change in understanding of the causes and management of alcohol problems to enable us to undertake this role. The three of us (two general practitioners and one psychologist) through our clinical work and research have been part of this change process.

Oxford
1988

P.D.A
P.W.
H.A.J.

Contents

1 Introduction 1
Alcohol and society 1
Relationship between consumption and damage 2
Alcohol and the general practitioner 4
2 How much people drink 6
Consumption trends 6
Who drinks what? 8
3 Why people drink 11
4 The drinking balance sheet 15
Drinking more—moving forwards on the continuum 15
Drinking less—moving backwards on the continuum 17
The general practitioner's role 18
5 Social harms related to alcohol 19
Who is at risk? 19
6 Psychological harms related to alcohol 21
Mood and the effects of conflict 22
Cognitive impairment 23
Drug use 23
7 Physical harms related to alcohol 24
Liver 25
Blood pressure and strokes 25
Cancer 26
Endocrine and sexual function 26
Pregnancy 27
Accidents 27
Alcohol and drugs 28

8 Risk and level of alcohol consumption 29
Who is at risk? 29
The importance of harm caused by moderate drinking 31
Alcohol and coronary heart disease 32

9 Measuring alcohol consumption 33
The need to measure 33
Measurement 34
Why use a questionnaire? 35
How to distribute a questionnaire 36
Identifying factors 37

10 Screening instruments: questionnaires and biological markers 38
Questionnaires 38
Alcohol meters 39
Biological markers 41

11 Management of different risk levels of alcohol consumption 43
Classification 43
Vulnerability 43
Low consumption—'normal vulnerability' 44
Low consumption—'high vulnerability' 44
Intermediate consumption—'normal vulnerability' 45
Intermediate consumption—'high vulnerability' 45
High consumption 45

12 Minimal intervention 45
Who needs it? 45
Components 48
Record keeping 52

13 Assessment of alcohol consumption 52
Who needs to be assessed? 52
Alcohol problems check-list 53
How to assess 54

History taking 54
Examination 54
Investigations 54

14 Intervention with high-risk patients 55

Reducing consumption 55
Pre-understanding 56
Understanding 56
Action 56
Moving from understanding to action 56
Goals for change 57
How to change 57
The drinks diary 58
Useful tips 58
Maintaining reduced drinking 60
Preventing relapse 60
Psychological therapies 61
Working with the family 61
Referral sources 62

15 Detoxification 64

Who needs it? 64
Where can detoxification be carried out? 64
Detoxification drugs 64
Dosage 65
Vitamins 65
Family support 65

16 The effectiveness of intervention 66

Evidence about smoking 66
Evidence about drinking 67
The DRAMS scheme 67
General practitioner intervention: the MRC study on life-style and health 67
Counselling heavy drinkers on medical wards 68
Identification and intervention of heavy drinking in middle-aged men, Malmo, Sweden 69

17 Audit and research 70
Information and assessment 70
Practice behaviour 71
Outcome and results 71

18 Local responses 72
Provision of information 72
Media 72
Advertising 72
Licensing 73
Patient participation 73

19 Prevention responses at national level 74
How could a general reduction in alcohol consumption be achieved? 74
Price and fiscal policy 74
Licensing laws 75
Advertising 77
Health education 77
The policy participants 78
The drinks trade 78
The Government 78
Government departments concerned with alcohol 78
The health lobby 80

Appendix I: Further information for the primary health care team 81
Books, reports, courses 81
Journals 83
Addresses 84

Appendix II: Further reading for patients 85

Index 86

1 Introduction

Alcohol and society

Alcohol is the most popular and widely used psychoactive drug in the world. In many societies alcohol has been incorporated into the fabric of everyday life, with its use being an integral part of the most joyous and most distressing of human occasions (Douglas 1987). Alcohol is used as a stimulant, a tranquillizer, an anaesthetic, a celebrant, a medicine, a social lubricant, a religious symbol, a food, a fuel, and as an indicator of the transition from work to play.

Many of the reasons for using alcohol are good, because they are positive. However, some reasons are negative, and this is where problems can arise and where the benefits of alcohol use start moving into disadvantages of alcohol use.

In England and Wales three million adults are heavy drinkers, drinking at levels leading to detectable biochemical abnormalities (8 per cent of the total adult population).

In England and Wales 700 000 adults have serious problems related to alcohol (2 per cent of the total adult population).

Heavy drinkers have a mortality rate over twice that of the normal population (Popham *et al.* 1984). Estimates suggest around 30 000 deaths are due to alcohol each year in England and Wales compared with, for example, 100 000 deaths due to cigarette smoking and 2000 deaths due to cervical cancer.

The financial costs of alcohol in terms of lost production and costs to the medical and social services in caring for individuals with alcohol problems has been calculated at least £2000 million a year (Fig. 1).

Excessive consumption cost the health services £100 million a year, of which £1.51 million a year were costs to general practice (McDonnel and Maynard 1985).

One in five patients on admission to medical wards have problems related to alcohol (Jarman and Kellett 1979).

1. *The social cost to industry*	
a. Sickness absence	641.51
b. Housework services	42.23
c. Unemployment	144.74
d. Premature death	567.70
2. *The social cost to the National Health Service*	
a. Psychiatric hospitals, in-patient costs (alcoholic psychosis, alcohol dependence syndrome, non-dependent abuse of alcohol)	17.90
b. Non-psychiatric hospitals, in-patient costs (alcoholic psychosis, alcohol dependence syndrome, alcoholic cirrhosis, and liver disease)	7.87
c. Other alcohol related diseases in-patient costs	68.58
d. General practitioner visits	1.51
3. *Society's response to alcohol related problems*	
a. Expenditure by national alcohol bodies	0.55
b. Research	0.49
4. *The social cost of material damage*	
a. Road traffic accidents (damage)	89.20
5. *The social cost of criminal activities*	
a. Police involvement in traffic offences (excluding road traffic accidents)	4.54
b. Police involvement in road traffic accidents (includes judiciary and insurance administration)	11.89
c. Drink-related court cases	15.79
Total (including unemployment and premature death)	**£1614.50m**
Total (excluding unemployment and premature death)	**£902.06m**

Fig. 1.1. Total resource costs of alcohol misuse, England and Wales, 1983 prices (£m).

Relationship between consumption and damage

It is accepted that national alcohol consumption is related to the level of alcohol related harm (Fig. 1.2).

The relationship between alcohol consumption and cirrhosis mortality is clearly established (Fig. 1.3).

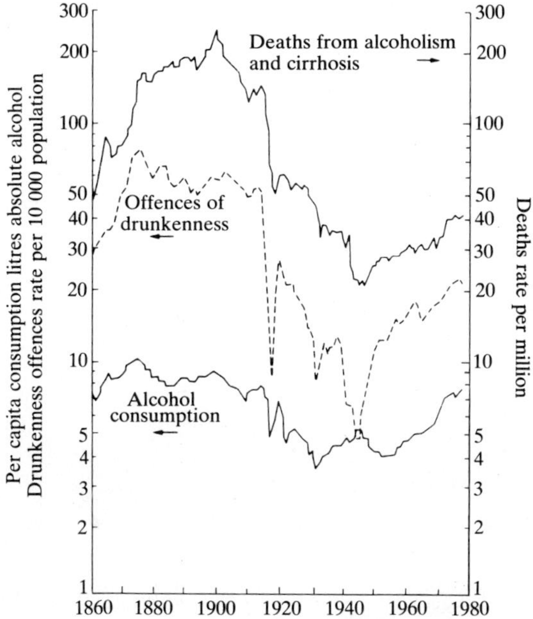

Fig. 1.2. Deaths from alcoholism and cirrhosis. Offences for drunkenness and consumption of alcohol, England and Wales, 1860–1978.

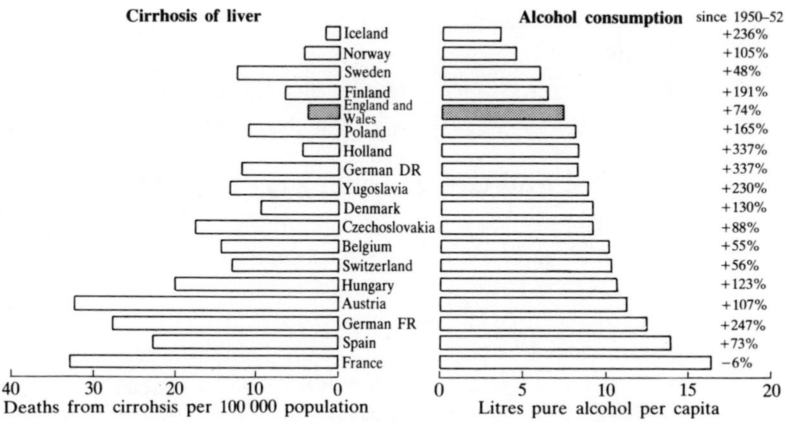

Fig. 1.3. Alcohol consumption and cirrhosis death rates. Selected countries.

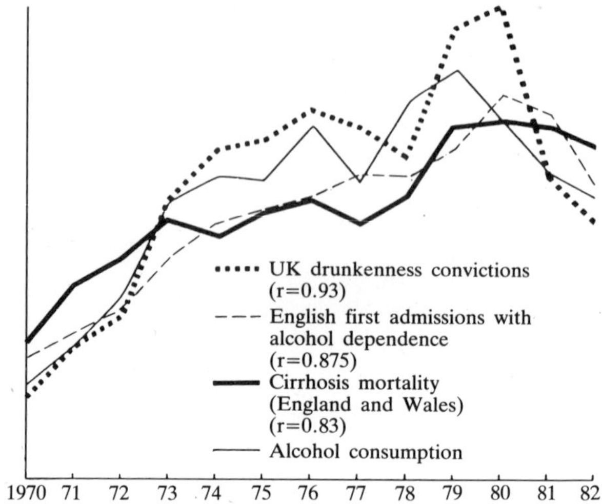

Fig. 1.4. Alcohol consumption, drunkenness convictions, alcoholism mortality (all per person aged 15 or over), 1970–82.

Furthermore, when alcohol consumption decreases so do the number of problems.

When, in the years 1981–82 for the first time in post-war Britain, consumption of alcohol per head fell temporarily from 10.4 litres of pure alcohol per adult to 9.2 litres (Fig. 1.4), there was an associated 11 per cent reduction in convictions for drunkenness, an 8 per cent fall in drinking and driving convictions, and a 4 per cent fall in deaths from liver cirrhosis (Kendell 1984).

Alcohol and the general practitioner

Every general practitioner has patients suffering from the harmful effects of alcohol. In this guideline we endeavour to present a constructive view of how the harms which arise from the use of alcohol result from its properties and the level and duration of consumption. A population suffers less ill-health and enjoys more well-being as its alcohol consumption decreases.

The first section of the book examines how much people drink, and their reasons for drinking. Information is then given on the social, psychological, and physical harms due to alcohol as they apply to general practice.

The second section of the book provides guidance on how alcohol consumption may be ascertained both for the practice population and for individual patients, and describes how individual assessment may be undertaken when consumption is found to be excessive.

The third section of the book contains advice on management of the heavy drinker. This includes a scheme of minimal intervention for those whose consumption poses a moderate risk and more intensive intervention for those whose consumption poses a major risk.

The fourth section of the book considers our involvement in general practice in the prevention of alcohol problems on a national and a local level, and the final section discusses how we may evaluate and audit the work that we are doing.

References

Douglas, M. (ed.) (1987). *Constructive drinking. Perspectives on drink from anthropology.* Cambridge University Press, Cambridge.

Jarman, C.M.B. and Kellett, J.M. (1979). Alcoholism in the General Hospital. *British Medical Journal,* **2,** 469–72.

Kendell, R.E. (1984). The beneficial consequences of the United Kingdom's declining per capital consumption of alcohol in 1979–82. *Alcohol and Alcoholism,* **19,** 271–6.

McDonnel, R. and Maynard, A. (1985). The costs of alcohol misuse. *British Journal of Addiction,* **80,** 27–35.

Popham, R.E., Schmidt, W. and Israelstam, S. (1984). Heavy alcohol consumption and physical health problems. In: *Research advances in alcohol and drug problems,* Vol. 8, (eds R.G. Smart, H. Capell, P. Glaser, Y. Israel, H. Kalant, W. Schmidt and J. Sellers), pp. 149–82, Plenum Publishing Corporation, New York.

2 How much people drink

Consumption trends

The adult population of the UK drank about twice as much alcohol in 1984 as it did in 1950. The increase in consumption is related to the price of alcohol which in real terms related to disposable income, almost halved between 1950 and 1984 (Fig. 2.1). Within this overall pattern of increase, spirit consumption increased by 135 per cent, wine consumption by more than 250 per cent, and beer by relatively less at 40 per cent (Fig. 2.2). There was a temporary dip in consumption after 1979 which was associated with the recession. In 1986, the British population drank the equivalent of over nine pints of beer per week for each individual over the age of 16, and spent £11 434 million in doing so. This represented 7.5 per cent of all

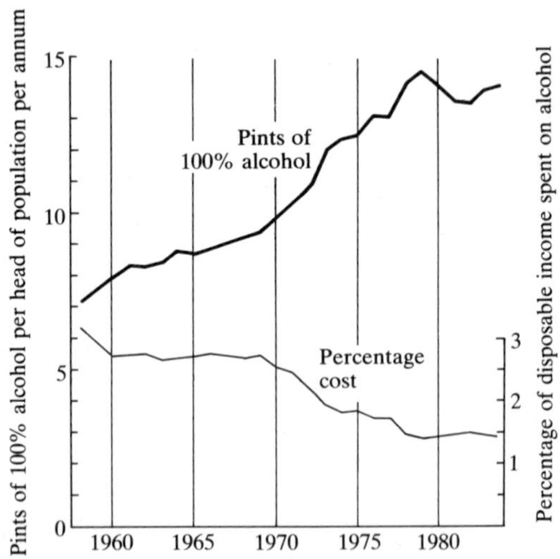

Fig. 2.1. Cost of alcohol as a percentage of personal disposable income, 1960–80.

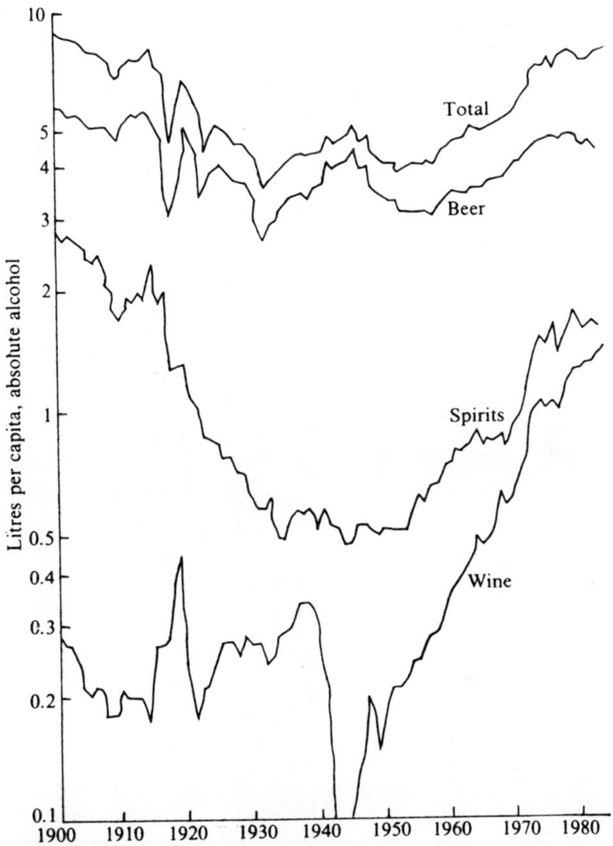

Fig. 2.2. Alcohol consumption by type, UK, 1900–84.

consumer expenditure and was more than that spent on clothing (£10 131 million) or on running cars (£10 150 million).

The present increase in alcohol consumption started from an historical low point in the period 1930–60, and there have been periods of much higher consumption. In the 1680s, for instance, beer consumption apparently reached an estimated peak level of 2.3 pints per person per day (including children), four times the present level.

Who drinks what?

Knowledge of current drinking patterns in the general population is derived largely from surveys in which people provide reports of their own consumption. The results should be treated with some caution as taxation figures show national consumption to be considerably more than that estimated in self-reporting surveys (Pernanen 1974).

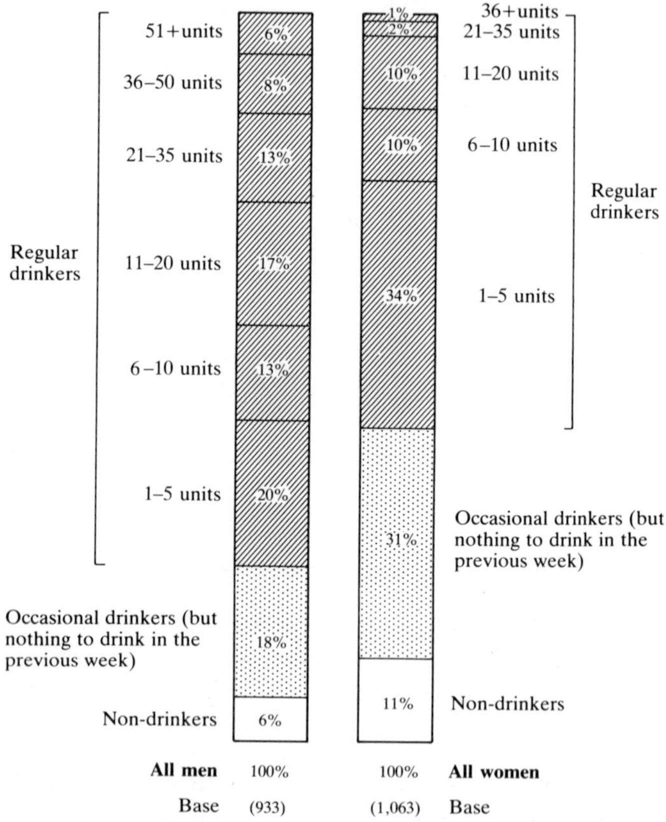

Fig. 2.3. Average weekly consumption of drinkers by sex and age, 1978.

Nevertheless, the results of these surveys can be taken as evidence of the variability in drinking habits in the population, and of the major differences between the sexes and between people of different ages.

Figures 2.3 and 2.4 are taken from Wilson's (1980*a*) survey which provides one of the most reliable sources of data on drinking

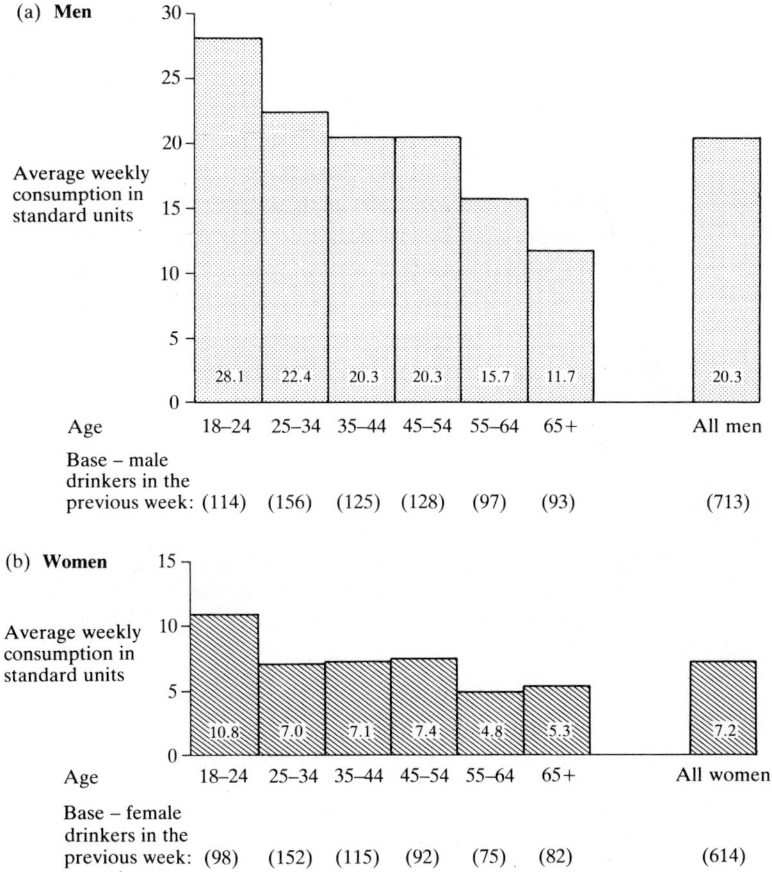

Fig. 2.4. Distribution of alcohol consumed in the previous week for men and women, 1978.

patterns in England and Wales. These results are based on detailed questioning about drinking during the week before interview.

There does not appear to be any consistent variation in overall alcohol consumption between social class groups in the UK, although there may be differences in the way consumption is distributed across days of the week.

Prevalence studies show that people who are unemployed drink more but there is no evidence to show that becoming unemployed itself 'leads' to heavy drinking (Iversen and Klausen 1981).

Many studies of alcohol problems have shown regional variations with higher figures in the north of England and Scotland than in the south. Part of the difference can probably be attributed to differences in detection, recording, and provision of services. There are, however, differences in drinking patterns; there is some evidence of greater 'binge' drinking in Scotland where 40 per cent of adult male drinkers had drunk more than eight units in one day, compared with 27 per cent in England (Wilson 1980*b*).

References

Iversen, L. and Kalusen, H. (1981). *Lukvingen af Nordhaus-Vaerflet.* Publication 13. Institut fur Social Medicin, Kobehavns Universitet.

Pernanen, K. (1974). Validity of survey data on alcohol use. In: Research Advances in Alcohol and Drug Problems. Vol. 1, (ed. R.J. Gibbons, Y. Israel, H. Kalant, R.E. Popham, W. Schmidt, and R.G. Smart), pp. 355–74.

Wilson, P. (1980*a*). *Drinking in England and Wales,* HMSO, London.

Wilson, P. (1980*b*). Drinking Habits in the United Kindom, *Population Trends,* **22,** 14–18.

3 Why people drink

To feel more relaxed in company
Because it goes well with meals
To make me feel more relaxed
To pick me up when I feel tired
To help me go to sleep
To relieve a stressful situation
Only because I'm offered a drink
I like the taste
To relieve a sense of boredom
To quench my thirst
To forget personal problems
To relieve a hangover
To have a good laugh
To feel good
To get drunk

Because it's the custom
For no reason
To reduce threats to feelings of inadequacy
To protect against depression
To relieve dependency conflict
To express rebellion against parents or other authority figures
To ease the tensions of an unhappy home life
To achieve peer status
To relieve stress in my job
To enhance fantasies of personal power
As self-reward
As sedation
To relieve sex role conflict

The length and variety of these lists, incomplete as they are, illustrate that alcohol is perceived to serve a wide variety of functions.

Because doctors deal with individual patients and because in the past they have focused mainly upon individual 'alcoholics', they have a strong inclination to regard risky and. harmful drinking as being determined by factors unique to a particular person or his or her particular personality.

The determinants of behaviour such as drinking, however, are as much social, cultural, and environmental as they are personal. Almost all surveys of the drinking behaviour of young people find that involvement in drinking is correlated with the behaviour of their friends (Orford 1985).

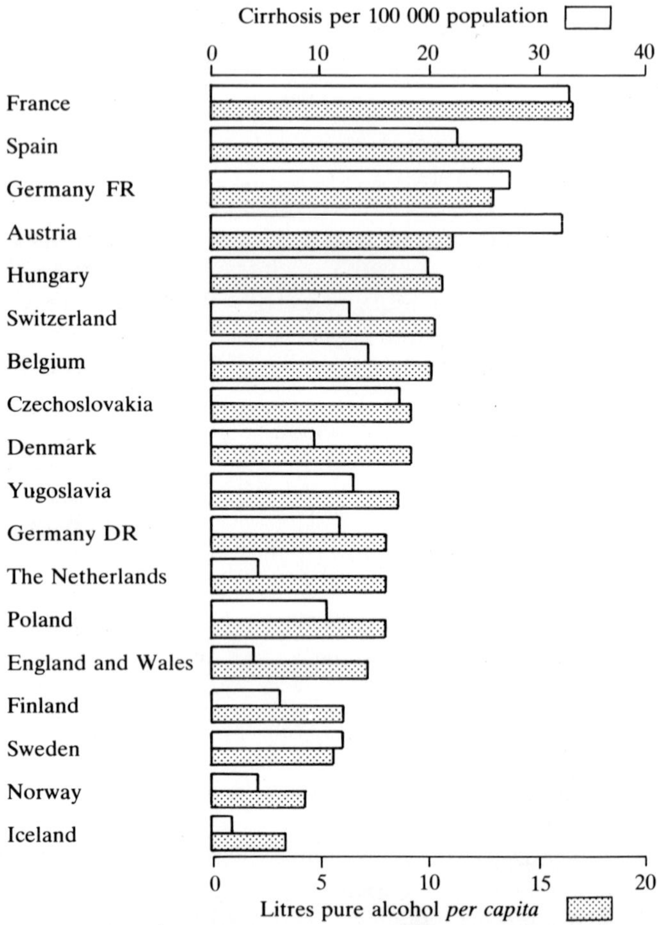

Fig. 3.1. Liver cirrhosis death rates and alcohol consumption in selected countries, mid-1970s. From Office of Health Economics (1981), reproduced with permission of the publisher.

The peer group appears to be the single most important determinant, at least of early drinking patterns in adolescence and young adulthood. The same is true of smoking and use of other drugs. Drinking is largely a social and recreational activity and it is therefore no surprise that friends have a major influence on drinking habits. This influence is not confined to young people.

Women in particular continue to be highly influenced by the drinking practices of their menfolk, and it is known that husbands of women who drink excessively or harmfully are likely to be heavy drinkers themselves (Jacob and Seilhamer 1982). Although excessive drinking may become a solitary affair for some people later on, drinking remains for most people and particularly for men, a social phenomenon throughout most of their drinking careers.

TABLE 3.1. Cirrhosis death rates by occupation

Occupational group rate	Standardized Mortality
Average occupation	100
Publicans	1017
Deck, engine room hands, bargemen, lightermen, boatmen	873
Barmen	612
Deck, engineering and radio officers, and pilots, ship	417
Electrical engineers (so described)	387
Hotel and residential club managers	342
Innkeepers	315
Fishermen	296
Chefs, cooks	265
Restauranteurs	263
Authors, writers, journalists	261
Drivers' mates	225
Winders, reelers	202
Other domestic and school helpers	141
Garage proprietors	140
Medical practitioners	115
Farm workers	45
Printing machine minders and assistants	32
Managers in building and contracting	22

Source: Office of Population Censuses and Surveys (1986).

It is more the rule than the exception to find in the drinking histories of excessive drinkers that some period has been spent living or working in an environment where alcohol was more than usual readily available and where heavy drinking was the norm.

Environments can be risky for the individuals who inhabit them, e.g. living in France carries a higher risk of cirrhosis of the liver than living in Norway (Fig. 3.1).

Entering adulthood in the early years of this century was more risky than immediately after the Second World War in Britain. Being brought up in England by first generation Irish immigrants is riskier than being brought up by 'native' English parents. Working in a brewery or public house is riskier than being a farm worker (Table 3.1).

People are subject to a variety of individual and social factors which influence their disposition to drink.

In recent years, awareness has also grown that hazardous drinking is not just a matter of individual psychology, pharmacology or occupation but it is also a public health matter (WHO 1980). There is a strong correlation between national consumption of alcohol and death rates from cirrhosis of the liver. There is also a strong inverse relationship between the relative price of alcohol and national alcohol consumption.

A study in Edinburgh showed that average alcohol consumption decreased following an increase in the price of alcohol in the 1981 budget (Kendell *et al.* 1983). The most important finding was that the heavy and suspected dependent drinkers reduced their consumption as much as the moderate consumers.

References

Jacob, T. and Seilhamer, R.A. (1982). The impact of spouses and how they can cope. In: *Alcohol and the family* (ed. J. Orford and J. Harwin), Croom Helm, London.

Kendell, R., De-Romaine, M. and Ritson, B. (1983). Effect of economic changes on Scottish drinking habits 1978–1982. *British Journal of Addiction,* **78,** 365–79.

Office of Population Censuses and Surveys (1986). *Occupational Mortality 1979–80, 1982–83*, Series DS, No. 6, Office of Population Censuses and Surveys, London.

Orford, J. (1985). Excessive appetites. *A psychological view of addictions.* John Wiley, Chichester.

(WHO) World Health Organization (1980). *Problems related to alcohol consumption.* Technical Report Series 650. WHO, Geneva.

4 The drinking balance sheet

The term 'alcoholism' has, for many years, offered the only framework for understanding harmful drinking. Although many illnesses are related to alcohol consumption we do not subscribe to the view that 'alcoholism' is in itself a disease.

Rather, the framework proposed in this guideline sees drinking distributed within a continuum from harm-free at one end to harmful drinking at the other. An individual's drinking behaviour is learned and shaped by experience and will be determined at any given stage by a balance of the advantages and disadvantages of the resultant pleasures and harms (Figs 4.1 and 4.2).

Everyone, whatever their current level of drinking has the choice to move in either direction within this continuum. Studies have shown that in many cases formerly heavy drinkers can resume lighter drinking at an acceptable level of risk (Vaillant 1983).

Drinking more—moving forwards on the continuum

Human beings are subject to change and development during a lifetime. Behaviour such as drinking does not occur in isolation but as part of a constellation of changing beliefs, preferences, and habits. Drinking behaviour cannot be divorced from the demands, both biological and social, of particular stages in the life cycle. Plant's (1979) study of the drinking habits of employees in the drinks trade demonstrates this. Plant was interested to know whether the risk of being employed in this trade was the result of self-selection of already heavy drinkers to this working environment or because of factors inherent in the job. It turned out to be both. As a group, people who enter such employment are heavy drinkers, but they become even heavier drinkers once they are in the work.

Another factor which may influence the development of excessive or risky drinking is the process of certain behaviour being

	Pay-offs from drinking	
	Positive	Negative
Feelings	'High', stimulated after a few drinks	Headache, dry mouth and mildly depressed next morning if drunk a lot
Performance	Increased energy and motivation immediately after lunch	Reduced concentration at work in afternoon if drink at lunchtime
Relationships with others	Closer, less tense with work colleagues	–
Economic	–	Leaves money short at weekend if drinks a lot Friday night
Others	Part of enjoyable relaxation at snooker club and at home with family and friends	–

Fig. 4.1. Hypothetical balance sheet of a moderate drinker.

	Pay-offs from drinking	
	Positive	Negative
Feelings	Helps cope with family and job worries, relaxes	Feel guilty about drinking so much
Performance	Can face working after a few drinks	Making mistakes at work. One or two near misses in car
Relationships with others	Meet several other heavy drinkers in local who are good company, able to assert myself	Family complaining not seeing me much, have embarrassed them a few times, they say I'm a changed character after drinking
Economic	–	Can't afford what I'm spending on drink
Others	–	Put on a lot of weight

Fig. 4.2. Hypothetical balance sheet of a heavy drinker.

rewarded or 'reinforced'. Behaviour which is rewarded sufficiently often becomes habitual and difficult to break. This process is aided by 'conditioning' whereby stimuli such as the sight and sounds of a public house, the smell of a favourite tipple, and everything associated with a pleasant drinking occasion takes on emotionally positive connotations.

These processes in combination are immensely powerful. As one writer put it: '*Never underestimate the strength of a habit*' (Reinhert 1968).

Drinking less—moving backwards on the continuum

The financial burden of drinking heavily may cause the drinker to cut back on drinking. The role of the family in moderating drinking cannot be overemphasized. The family plays a major part in helping or hindering a reduced level of drinking. By encouraging excessive drinking or by unknowingly contributing to a spiral of increased family tension a family may make it more difficult to reduce drinking. On the other hand, the family may be the principal force for change by influencing one of its members towards moderate drinking and by providing care and affection.

Finally, medical advice relating physical ill-health such as gastritis and overweight to over-drinking may help a patient to understand the need to take immediate corrective action.

The general practitioner's role

It is within this framework of a balance of advantages and disadvantages resulting from drinking and of a continuum along which an individual may move at different stages of the life cycle that the general practitioner's role should be considered. As one uniquely well placed and qualified to detect the signs of risky and harmful drinking and to influence those who are drinking excessively, the general practitioner has a crucial role to play—we are in a strong and privileged position to influence our patients' drinking habits for good.

References

Plant, M.A. (1979). *Drinking careers.* Tavistock, London.

Reinert, R. (1968). The concept of alcoholism as a bad habit. *Bulletin of the Menninger Clinic,* **32,** 35–46.

Vaillant, G. (1983). *The natural history of alcoholism.* Harvard University Press, London.

5 Social harms related to alcohol

Alcohol related disabilities may be considered, for convenience, under three headings: social, psychological, and physical. In reality an individual's experience may involve a clustering of these types of difficulties.

Who is at risk?

Traditional concepts separating 'alcoholics' from the rest of the drinking population have now been replaced by a view that drinking and related problems occur within a continuum. *Any alcohol user is at risk* of problems and generally the more alcohol consumed the greater the risk.

We are familiar with this concept in the case of blood pressure and serum cholesterol, both of which are risk factors for coronary heart disease. They are distributed within a continuum; the higher the level of either, the greater the risk of developing the disease.

Although there is a high proportion of problems among heavy drinkers, their contribution to the total number of problems in the country is small. *The majority of alcohol-related problems in society are contributed by the larger numbers of light and moderate drinkers.* This phenomenon, common to all risk factors of this kind (including blood pressure and serum cholesterol), is sometimes known as the 'prevention paradox' and is of crucial importance in considering strategies for prevention.

There are two aspects of alcohol-related disabilities producing social harms relating to *intoxication* and *regular, heavy consumption.*

Social problems relating to intoxication

Family arguments
Domestic violence
Criminal damage
Theft

Child neglect/abuse	Burglary
Domestic accidents	Assault
Absenteeism from work	Homicide
Accidents at work	Drinking and driving
Inefficient work	Taking cars and driving away
Public drunkenness	Road traffic accidents
Public aggression	Sexually deviant acts
Football hooliganism	Unwanted pregnancy

Social problems relating to regular, heavy drinking

Family problems	Fraud
Divorce	Debt
Homelessness	Vagrancy
Work difficulties	Habitual convictions for drunkenness
Unemployment	
Financial difficulties	

The idea of social disability implies failure of an individual to perform adequately in any role expected of him or her. It also includes behaviour which transgresses social rules, for example, crime or sexual deviance.

Social disability is thus highly dependent on social norms. These norms may be different for men and women, for different age groups, between social classes, and between countries.

Both intoxication and regular heavy drinking are associated with a wide range of problems involving, for example, the family, employment, crime, and drinking and driving offences.

Children are especially at risk. Neglect and child abuse are related to intoxication and regular heavy drinking (Nylander 1960; Orme and Rimmer 1981). Excessive drinking is a frequent cause of marital problems and divorce.

There are strong links between alcohol and crime. Among prisoners in England and Wales about 50 per cent to 66 per cent of the men and 15 per cent of the women have a serious problem related to alcohol.

A study showed that between 10 p.m. and 2 a.m., 93 per cent of all arrested persons were intoxicated (Jeffs and Saunders 1983). In the

[Ph]ysical harms related to alcohol

[P]hysical harm also relates separately to intoxication and to regular, [h]eavy consumption.

Intoxication and Physical Problems

Hepatitis	Strokes
Gastritis	Acute alcohol poisoning
Pancreatitis	Failure to take prescribed medication
Gout	Impotence
Cardiac arrythmia	Fetal damage
Accidents	
Trauma	

Regular, heavy drinking, and physical problems

Obesity	Reactions with other drugs
Diabetes	Fatty liver
Cardiomyopathy	Hepatitis
Raised blood pressure	Cirrhosis
Strokes	Liver cancer
Brain damage	Gastritis
Neuropathy	Pancreatitis
Myopathy	Cancer of mouth, larynx, oesophagus
Sexual dysfunction	Cancer of breast
Infertility	Cancer of colon (?)
Fetal damage	Nutritional deficiencies
Haemopoietic toxicity	

The physical harms related to alcohol are widespread and involve all aspects of work in general practice. It is of particular importance in the management of chronic conditions such as diabetes and raised blood pressure.

period 1952–83, when consumption of alcohol in the UK increased by 89 per cent, convictions for drunkenness rose from 12 per 1000 population to 29 per 1000.

In the period 1960–84 drink driving offences rose from 23 900 to 98 000. It is recognized that these figures reflect the degree of police activity as well as the amount of drinking. However, at least one study has shown that on a given evening a quarter of all men and one in 13 of all women drink sufficient alcohol to put their blood alcohol level above the legal limit (80 mg per 100 ml) (Wilson 1980). The strong association between raised gamma-GT activity and accidents in drivers over the age of 30 indicates that a large proportion of these accidents involve heavy drinkers.

References

Jeffs, B. and Saunders, W. (1983). Minimising alcohol related offences by enforcement of existing licensing legislation. *British Journal of Addiction*, **78,** 67–77.

Nylander, I. (1960). Children of alcoholic fathers. *Acta Pediatrica Scandinavica*, **49,** suppl. 121.

Orme, T.C. and Rimmer, J. (1981). Alcohol and child abuse: a review. *Journal of Studies on Alcohol*, **42,** 273–87.

Wilson, P. (1980). *Drinking in England and Wales.* HMSO, London.

6 Psychological harms related to alcohol

Psychological harms also vary depending on whether they relate to intoxication or to regular heavy drinking.

Intoxication

Insomnia	Amnesia
Depression	Attempted suicide
Anxiety	Suicide

Regular, heavy drinking

Insomnia	Delerium Tremens
Depression	Withdrawal fits
Anxiety	Hallucinosis
Attempted suicide	Dementia
Suicide	Gambling
Changes in personality	Misuse of other drugs
Amnesia	

Acute intoxication is an example where physical, psychological, and social harms overlap.

Symptoms of intoxication typically include slurred speech and impairment of co-ordination, thinking, and memory. Respiratory depression and inhalation of vomit can kill.

Regular heavy drinking may produce more general cognitive impairment. Tolerance to some of these effects is acquired by regular, heavy consumption.

A blood alcohol level of 150–200 mg/100 ml may cause an inexperienced drinker to be intoxicated whilst a regular heavy drinker may appear to react normally with a blood alcohol of 500 mg/100 ml.

Mood and the effects of conflict

Although alcohol is frequently used to relieve unpleasant feelings such as anxiety and depression, there is evidence that persistent heavy drinking may actually exacerbate these feelings. This is just one of the many 'vicious circles' which may be set up as a result of drinking.

Another arises as a result of associated feelings of conflict and guilt. Guilt about behaviour produces a tendency to minimize its extent and the harm it is causing and to become more secretive. This is not an indication of a basic resistance to change but a natural psychological response to the distress the patient feels. Feelings of low self-esteem combined with anxiety, depression, and guilt contributes to the very high rate of attempted and successful suicides among heavy drinkers (Office of Health Economics 1981).

Cognitive impairment

'Morning-after' amnesia often ac
Frequent and more lasting per
serious risk or progressive damag

As many as half the heavy drinke
be shown to have significant disabi
despite apparently normal mental st
Age and drinking history increase the

Drug use

Heavy use of alcohol may be linked wi
hypnotics and other drugs, particularly in th
drugs such as doctor, nurses, and pharmacis

Young people may alternate between heav
amphetamines, cannabis or other fashionable
(Plant *et al.* 1985). Heavy smoking, drug use, and
tion are strongly associated.

References

Office of Health Economics (1981). *Alcohol—Reducing the*
Health Economics, London.

Plant, M.A., Peck, D.F., and Samuel, E. (1985). *Alcohol, drug*
leavers. Tavistock, London.

Thomson, A.D. and Ron, M.A. (1982). Alcohol-related brain dama
Medical Bulletin, **38,** 87–94.

7 P

Liver (Fig. 7.1)

Excess alcohol consumption can lead to the development of a wide spectrum of liver injury ranging from fatty liver, hepatitis, and cirrhosis to primary hepatocellular carcinoma.

Although only about 10–15 per cent of heavy drinkers develop cirrhosis, their mortality from this disease may be as much as 10 times higher than average. Liver function tests show severe impairment in 25 per cent and to a lesser degree in 50 per cent (see: Chapter 10, p. 42). It seems that alcohol provides a setting for potential liver damage and an additional factor is needed for the induction of cirrhosis.

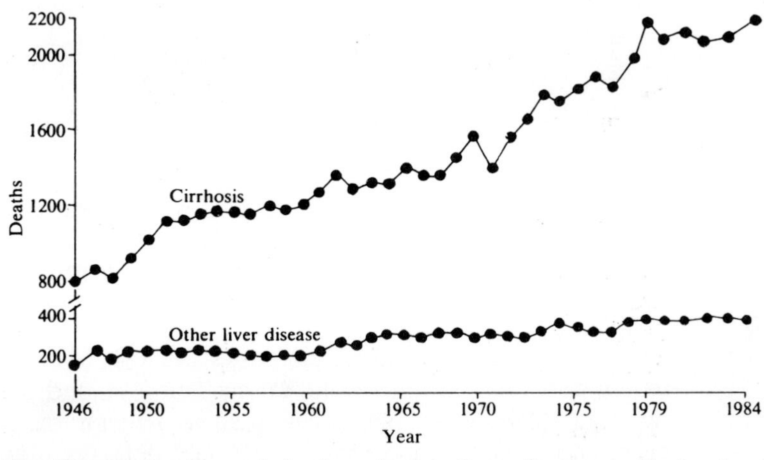

Fig. 7.1. Deaths from cirrhosis and other liver disease in England and Wales, 1946–84.

Blood pressure and strokes (Fig. 7.2)

There is a linear relationship between alcohol consumption and blood pressure that is independent of age, weight, and cigarette smoking (Klatsky *et al.* 1977).

Excess alcohol intake is probably the most common identifiable cause of raised blood pressure. Heavy drinkers have a two-fold increased risk of death from stroke.

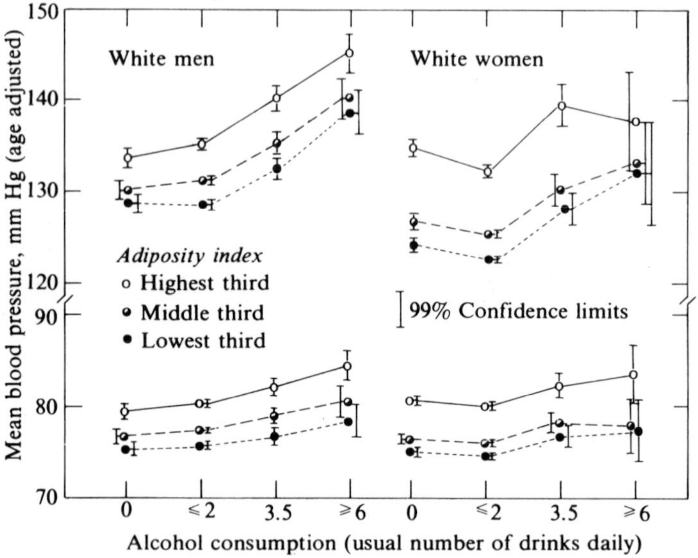

Fig. 7.2. Blood pressure related to alcohol consumption.

Cancer

Heavy alcohol consumption increases the risk of cancer of the mouth and pharynx three-fold, larynx four-fold, and oesophagus two-fold (MacSween 1982). The relative risk for cancer of the oesophagus may be increased to 150-fold in heavy drinkers who also smoke heavily. Heavy alcohol consumption may also be associated with an increased incidence of cancer of the colon and rectum (Schmidt and Popham 1981). There is substantial evidence that even moderate doses of alcohol constitute a risk factor for breast cancer in women (Willett *et al.* 1987).

Endocrine and sexual function

It is well known that intoxication leads to impotence and impairment of sexual performance.

Even moderate amounts of alcohol consumption (6 units per day) are related to impotence and male infertility.

Many heavy drinking women complain of sexual difficulty such as reduced responsiveness and of menstrual problems such as cycle irregularities and amenorrhea.

Pregnancy

Heavy alcohol intake in pregnancy is associated with a combination of fetal abnormalities including dysfunction of the central nervous system, growth deficiency, and abnormal facial characteristics (Jones *et al.* 1973). These abnormalities may occur in about one-third of the children born to mothers drinking the equivalent of half a bottle of whisky a day, i.e. up to 100 units per week, although affected children show considerable variation in the extent of severity of damage.

Moderate drinking (16–35 units per week) is associated with an increased risk of spontaneous abortion, still birth, congenital malformations, and growth retardation (Barrison *et al.* 1985). Very light drinking, i.e. less than 5 units per week, does not seem to have any harmful effect on fetal development.

Accidents

Excluding traffic accidents, nearly two-thirds of male admissions to accident and emergency facilities with head injuries have blood alcohol levels equivalent to having drunk six or more pints of beer (Murray 1977).

About one-third of home accidents are alcohol related and heavy drinkers have an accident rate at work three times higher than normal (Observer and Maxwell 1959).

Alcohol is the single most common factor in death by drowning.

In England and Wales it is estimated that alcohol intoxication is involved in the deaths of over 500 young people each year, i.e. about 10 per cent of all mortality of persons under 25 (Harvard 1977).

TABLE 7.1. The reaction between alcohol and commonly prescribed drugs

Drugs affected	Effect
Antihypertensives (2.5)	Potentiation
Warfarin, other coumarins (2.8)	Potentiation
Hypnotics, sedatives (4.1)	Potentiation
Tricyclic antidepressants (4.3)	Potentiation of sedative effect
Cephamandole, latamoxef, metronidazole (5.1)	Disulfiram reactions
Antidiabetic (oral and insulin) (6.1)	Potentiation
Metformin (6.1)	Increased risk of lactic acidosis
Chlorpropamide (6.1)	Flushing in susceptible patients
Procarbazine (8)	Disulfiram reaction
Monosulfiram (13)	Disulfiram reaction

Figures in brackets refer to paragraph numbers in the *British Natural Formulary*.

Source: British National Formulary (1987). Appendix 1, pp. 419–28.

Alcohol and drugs

There is an interaction between alcohol and many types of prescribed drugs (see Table 7.1).

References

Barrison, I.G., Waterson, E.J., and Murray-Lyon, I.M. (1985). Adverse effects of alcohol on pregnancy. *British Journal of Addiction*, **80,** 11–22.

British Medical Association and the Pharmaceutical Society of Great Britain. (1987). *British National Formulary*. No. 13, 419–20.

Harvard, J. (1977). Alcohol and road accidents. In *New knowledges and new responses* (ed. G. Edwards, and M. Grant). Croom Helm, London.

Jones, K.L. *et al.* (1973). Patterns of malformation in offspring of alcoholic mothers. *Lancet*, **1,** 1267–71.

Klatsky, A.L. *et al.* (1977). Alcoholic consumption and blood pressure. Kaiser—Permanente multiphasic health examination data. *New England Journal of Medicine*, **296,** 1194–1200.

MacSween, R.M.N. (1982). Alcohol and cancer. *British Medical Bulletin*, **38,** 31–3.

Murray, W.R. (1977). Head injuries and alcohol. In *Alcoholism: a new knowledge of new responses.* (ed. G. Edwards, and M. Grant). Croom Helm, London.

Observer and Maxwell, M.A. (1959). A study of absenteeism, accidents and sickness payments in problem drinkers in one industry. *Quarterly Journal of Studies on Alcohol,* **20,** 302–12.

Schmidt, W. and Popham, R.E. (1981). The role of drinking and smoking in mortality from cancer and other causes in male alcoholics. *Cancer,* **47,** 1031–41.

Willett, W.C. *et al.* (1987). Moderate alcohol consumption and the risk of breast cancer. *New England Journal of Medicine,* **36,** 1174–80.

8 Risk and levels of alcohol consumption

Many individuals want to know their personal risk from different levels of alcohol consumption and would like guidelines about sensible drinking. General practitioners therefore need a guide for action.

Who is at risk?

A number of authors have studied the relationship between consumption and damage. Pequignot *et al.* (1978) showed that men who consumed between 28 and 42 units[1] of alcohol a week had a risk of developing cirrhosis six times that of men with a weekly consump-

[1] 1 unit contains 8 g of alcohol and is equivalent to a half pint of beer, a glass of wine or sherry, or one pub measure of spirits.

tion of less than 14 units of alcohol a week. This risk increased to 14 times for men drinking between 42 and 56 units a week.

The Kaiser–Permanente study (Klatsky *et al.* 1977) demonstrated the direct relationship between alcohol consumption and blood pressure which was found to be independent of age, sex, weight, and cigarette smoking.

The UK Civil Servant Study (Marmot *et al.* 1981) demonstrated that men drinking 30 or more units of alcohol a week had twice the mortality rate at 10-year follow-up, compared with men drinking between 1 and 8 units a week.

Studies have shown that women may be more susceptible to the toxic effects of alcohol than men. Research strongly indicates that women who drink to excess risk have accelerated development of fatty liver, hepatitis, cirrhosis of the liver, obesity, anaemia, malnutrition, and gastro-intestinal haemorrhage compared to men (Hill 1984).

Heavy drinking in pregnancy is particularly hazardous and alcohol influences women differently at various times of the menstrual cycle.

At the extremes of youth and old age alcohol may also have disproportionate effects.

The following figures, which correspond with the recommendations of the Royal Colleges of General Practitioners, Physicians and Psychiatrists, represent a reasonable guide to personal risk at different levels of alcohol consumption.

Risk	*Women*	*Men*
Low	Less than 15 units per week	Less than 20 units per week
Moderate or Intermediate	15–35 units per week	20–50 units per week
High	36 units per week or more	51 units per week or more

Drinkers in the low category are unlikely to experience any long-term health risks from this level of consumption. However, if all their drinking took place in one or two bouts, then they are at an increased risk of an accident.

Those at the lower end of the moderate category, i.e. BELOW 21 UNITS PER WEEK FOR WOMEN AND BELOW 35 UNITS PER WEEK FOR MEN are unlikely to experience long term health risks *provided that their drinking is spread throughout the week.*

Those drinking at the upper end of the moderate category, i.e. AT LEAST 21 UNITS PER WEEK FOR WOMEN AND 35 UNITS PER WEEK FOR MEN are drinking at levels of consumption that are likely to damage their health.

Those drinking in the high category, i.e. ABOVE 35 UNITS PER WEEK FOR WOMEN AND ABOVE 50 UNITS PER WEEK FOR MEN are almost certainly already damaging their health.

It must be emphasized that whatever upper limit is set for low to moderate risk it cannot be assumed that anyone is necessarily safe below this level of consumption.

There are no safe limits—only guidelines.

The importance of harm caused by moderate drinking

The majority of alcohol-related problems in society are contributed by the relatively large numbers of light and moderate drinkers although only a small proportion of them individually have alcohol related problems. This concept is illustrated in Fig. 8.1.

Figure 8.1 shows the estimated effects on the reduction of mortality rates by reducing alcohol consumption to the next lower risk level. The highest impact occurs in the moderate drinks (11–35 units per week) whose mortality rates would fall by 90 per 10 000 population in a 10-year period.

Band	Units	Per cent of population in this band	10 yr death rate per 10 000 population	Death rate by reducing consumption to next lower band	Number of lives saved per 10 000 Pop. in 10 yr period if everyone reduces consumption in next lower band
1	1-10	60	600	600	—
2	11-35	30	900	600	90
3	36 +	10	1200	900	30

Fig. 8.1. Estimated effect on the reduction of mortality rates by reduction of level of alcohol consumption.

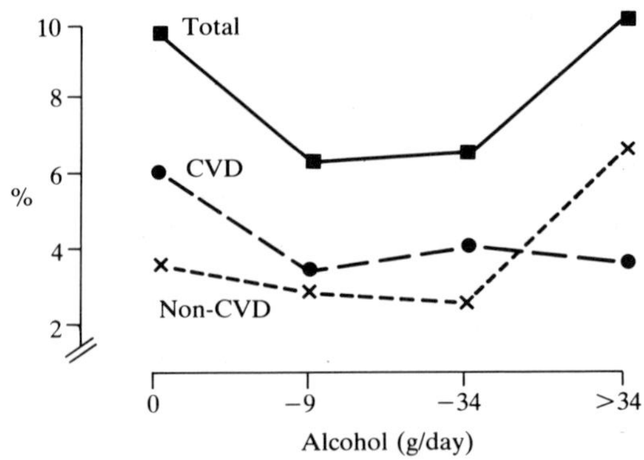

Fig. 8.2. Ten-year mortality (age-adjusted percentage) all causes, cardiovascular and non-cardiovascular according to daily alcohol consumption. From Marmot *et al.* (1981), reproduced by permission of the Editor.

Alcohol and coronary heart disease

A number of studies have demonstrated that low alcohol consumption (in the range of 1–2 units per day) is protective against coronary heart disease when compared to abstention (Marmot, 1984) and Fig. 8.2. This relationship remains when individuals who are abstaining because of ill health are excluded from the analysis. The exact mechanism of the effect remains uncertain.

The finding does not alter the public health message which states that overall there is a direct relationship between alcohol consumption and harm.

References

Hill, S.Y. (1984). Vulnerability and the biomedical consequence of alcoholism and alcohol related problems among women. In *Alcohol problems in women* (ed. S.C. Witsnack and L. Beckman), pp. 120–54, Guildford Press, New York.

Klatsky, A.L. *et al.* (1977). Alcohol consumption and blood pressure, Kaiser–Permanente multiphasic health examination data. *New England Journal of Medicine*, **296,** 1194–1200.

Marmot, M. (1984). Alcohol and coronary heart disease. *International Journal of Epidemiology*, **13,** 160–7.

Marmot, M. G. *et al.* (1981). Alcohol and Mortality: a U-shaped curve. *Lancet*, **1,** 580–3.

Pequignot, G., Tuyns, A.J., and Berta, J.L. (1978). Ascitic cirrhosis in relation to alcohol consumption. *International Journal of Epidemiology*, **7,** 113–20.

9 Measuring alcohol consumption

The need to measure

As we have already said, alcohol consumption acts as a risk factor in much the same way as blood pressure. As each increases so does the likelihood of damage. Lowering consumption of alcohol, or similarly the level of blood pressure, substantially reduces morbidity and mortality.

Helping to reduce the risk even by a small amount in the great majority of the population whose consumption is at low or intermediate levels will have a major impact on the overall health of the community.

Expectations from the public of advice from general practitioners about healthy living are rising and doctors are seen to have responsibility for knowing about and advising on potentially damaging factors in personal life-style (Wallace and Haines 1985; Skinner *et al.* 1985).

Thus, general practices need to recognize that an attitude of preventive care towards their patients' alcohol consumption is both valid and necessary.

As doctors become more involved in preventive medicine, detection of risk from harm from alcohol becomes just one of a number of areas of concern—exercise diet and weight, smoking and drugs, stress and pollution are all perceived as legitimate topics for enquiry. Ideally, each practice will establish a plan for finding out about every patient's alcohol consumption and placing each one in a category depending upon current drinking. A system should be developed for recording and assessing this information, and for acting upon it.

Measurement

Measuring blood pressure poses no problem; the sphygmomanometer is easy to use and highly reliable. However, there is no equivalent in the case of alcohol consumption, and many doctors find taking a drinking history difficult and unrewarding. Many are cautious about asking direct questions about alcohol, perhaps believing that such questions will not be well received or that if alcohol is an important factor the patient will lie and evade the issue.

This impression probably derives from experience with patients with major alcohol-related problems and/or dependence who frequently display considerable denial. However, there is good evidence (Duffy and Waterton 1984; Poikalainen 1985) that information which most patients provide is sufficiently truthful.

Why use a questionnaire?

Systematic measurement by a questionnaire (Fig. 9.1–9.2) is more useful than just asking a patient: 'How much do you drink?' Responses are likely to be vague: 'Not very much'; 'I'm a social drinker'; 'A lot at weekends'.

HERE ARE SOME QUESTIONS ABOUT THINGS YOU MAY DO WHICH MIGHT AFFECT YOUR HEALTH

Please answer ALL the questions
Just CIRCLE the answer which you think most nearly applies to you
Please Circle only ONE answer for each question

1. **IN THE LAST MONTH: have you smoked any cigarettes?** YES NO

If YES:
About how many cigarettes have you smoked a day

1-4	5-14	15-24	25 or more

2. **IN THE LAST MONTH: have you had an alcoholic drink at all?** YES NO

If YES: Please answer A and B
A. About how often have you had any of the following types of drink over the last month

Beer, lager, cider, etc	not at all	less than once a week	1-2 times a week	3-4 times a week	5-6 times a week	Every day
wine, sherry, vermouth etc	not at all	less than once a week	1-2 times a week	3-4 times a week	5-6 times a week	Every day
gin, vodka, rum, brandy, whisky, etc	not at all	less than once a week	1-2 times a week	3-4 times a week	5-6 times a week	Every day

B. When you've had a drink over the last month how much of the following types of drink have you usually had a day (i.e. 24 hour period)

Pints of beer, lager cider etc	none	½-1	1-2	3	4-5	6-7	8 or more
Glasses of wine, sherry vermouth etc	none	1-2	3-4	5-6	7-9	11-14	15 or more
Measures of spirits (gin, vodka rum, brandy, whisky etc)	none	1-2	3-4	5-6	7-9	11-14	15 or more

3. **IN THE LAST MONTH: have you been dieting to lose weight** YES NO

If YES:
How many pounds have you managed to lose?

0	1-3	4-7	8 or more

4 **IN THE LAST MONTH: have you been exercising to get fit to keep fit?** YES NO

If YES:
On average, how many days per week have you been exercising?

1-2	3-4	5-6	Every dav

And, on average, how many minutes per day have you been exercising?

1-14	15-29	30-44	45 or more

Fig. 9.1. An example of a questionnaire concerning general health.

ALCOHOL MEASUREMENT CARD

On average how many days a week do you have a drink of alcohol? ☐

On average, on a day when you have had a drink, how much have you usually had?

half pints of beer, cider	glasses of wine, sherry	singles of spirits	TOTAL
☐	☐	☐	☐

Alcohol consumption per week (Number of days X quantity) ☐

Name________________ Date________________

Fig. 9.2. Alcohol measurement card.

The Frequency/Quantity scale on the questionnaire will tell you:

1. How often the patient drinks.

2. How much he/she drinks on each occasion.

Multiplying one by the other gives an accurate estimate of weekly alcohol consumption.

How to distribute the questionnaire

Here are some suggestions:

1. Each new patient registering at the practice can be handed a copy of the questionnaire to complete and return.

2 Receptionists can put a copy of the questionnaire into the notes of patients as they attend for surgery. The patients can then be handed a copy to complete when they check in at the desk for their appointment.

3 A supply of questionnaires can be kept in the doctor's surgery or nurse's room. One can be given to each patient during the consultation.

Identifying factors

Some patients are particularly likely to be heavy drinkers. These include:

1. Patients with high blood pressure.

2. Patients who are overweight.

Other associated factors are:

(1) patients with a history of recurrent injuries or accidents;

(2) patients with non-specific gastro-intestinal complaints;

(3) patients with marital problems or a history of absenteeism;

(4) patients with a history of anxiety/depression;

(5) patients with high risk occupations;

(6) those with early signs of harm (e.g. abnormal liver function tests); or

(7) those with a strong family history of drinking.

References

Duffy, J.C., and Waterton, J.J. (1984). Under-reporting of alcohol consumption in sample surveys: The effect of computer interviewing in field work. *British Journal of Addiction,* **79,** 303–8.

Poikalainen, K. (1985). Underestimation of recalled alcohol intake in relation to actual consumption. *British Journal of Addiction,* **80,** 215–6.

Skinner, H.A. *et al.* (1985). Lifestyle assessment: Just asking makes a difference. *British Medical Journal,* **290,** 214–6.
Wallace, P. and Haines, A. (1985). Use of a questionnaire in general practice to increase the recognition of patients with excessive alcohol consumption. *British Medical Journal,* **290,** 1949–53.

10 Screening instruments: Questionnaires and biological markers

Questionnaires

Chapter 9 discussed the use of quantity frequency questionnaires in eliciting information about alcohol intake. Questionnaires may also be used for identifying individuals suffering psychosocial consequences because of their drinking. Of the numerous questionnaires available the brief MAST (Fig. 10.1) and the CAGE (Fig. 10.2) have been used most. In its original study, using a cut-off score of 6 and above, the brief MAST identified all of 60 alcoholics and gave a false-positive rate of seven out of 62 non-alcoholics (Pokorny *et al.* 1972). Eighty-one per cent of known alcoholics answered positively to two or more of the CAGE questionnaires, compared with 11 per cent of non-alcholics (Mayfield *et al.* 1974). Although both instruments have performed well in clinic settings, in general practice and community settings, they have failed to detect approximately half those individuals who are known to be at risk (Saunders and Kershaw 1980). They are therefore of limited usefulness.

In 1987, the World Health Organization (Saunders and Aarland 1987) developed a 'core' screening instrument for screening persons with early signs of alcohol-related problems (Figs 10.3 and 10.4). The maximum possible score is 40. Using a cut-off point of a

Questions	Circle correct answers	
1. Do you feel you are a normal drinker?	Yes (0)	No (2)
2. Do friends or relatives think you are a normal drinker?	Yes (0)	No (2)
3. Have you ever attended a meeting of Alcoholics Anonymous (AA)?	Yes (5)	No (0)
4. Have you ever lost friends or girlfriends/boyfriends because of drinking?	Yes (2)	No (0)
5. Have you ever gotten into trouble at work because of drinking?	Yes (2)	No (0)
6. Have you ever neglected your obligations, your family, or your work for two or more days in a row because you were drinking?	Yes (2)	No (0)
7. Have you ever had delirium tremens (DTs), severe shaking, heard voices or seen things that weren't there heavy drinking?	Yes (2)	No (0)
8. Have you ever gone to anyone for help about your drinking?	Yes (5)	No (0)
9. Have you ever been in a hospital because of drinking?	Yes (5)	No (0)
10. Have you ever been arrested for drunk driving or driving after drinking?	Yes (2)	No (0)

Fig. 10.1. The brief MAST.

1. Have you ever felt you should *cut* down on your drinking?
2. Have people *annoyed* you by criticizing your drinking?
3. Have you ever felt bad or *guilty* about your drinking?
4. Have you ever had a drink first thing in the morning to steady your nerves or get rid of a hangover (eye-opener)?

Fig. 10.2. The CAGE questionnaire.

score of 10 in community settings the instrument accurately identified 80 per cent of individuals at risk because of their drinking. The instrument had a false-positive rate of 11 per cent. A positive finding had a predictive value of 60 per cent and a negative finding a predictive value of 95 per cent (Saunders and Aarland 1987).

Alcohol meters

Alcohol meters cost about £250, and measure the breath ethanol concentration. They are essentially the same as those used by the police in roadside checks. The one major study of their use in

Please circle the answer that is correct for you.

1. How often do you have a drink* containing alcohol?

NEVER	MONTHLY OR LESS	TWO TO FOUR TIMES A MONTH	TWO TO THREE TIMES A WEEK	FOUR OR MORE TIMES A WEEK

2. How many drinks containing alcohol do you have on a typical day when you are drinking?

1 OR 2	3 OR 4	5 OR 6	7 – 9	10 OR MORE

3. How often do you have six or more drinks on one occasion?

NEVER	LESS THAN MONTHLY	MONTHLY	WEEKLY	DAILY OR ALMOST DAILY

4. How often during the last year have you found it difficult to get the thought of alcohol out of your mind?

NEVER	LESS THAN MONTHLY	MONTHLY	WEEKLY	DAILY OR ALMOST DAILY

5. How often during last year have you found you were not able to stop drinking once you had started?

NEVER	LESS THAN MONTHLY	MONTHLY	WEEKLY	DAILY OR ALMOST DAILY

6. How often during the last year have you been unable to remember what happened the night before because you had been drinking?

NEVER	LESS THAN MONTHLY	MONTHLY	WEEKLY	DAILY OR ALMOST DAILY

7. How often during the last year have you needed a first drink in the morning to get yourself going after a heavy drinking session?

NEVER	LESS THAN MONTHLY	MONTHLY	WEEKLY	DAILY OR ALMOST DAILY

8. How often during the last year have you had a feeling of guilt or remorse after drinking?

NEVER	LESS THAN MONTHLY	MONTHLY	WEEKLY	DAILY OR ALMOST DAILY

9. Have you or someone else been injured as a result of your drinking?

No	YES BUT NOT IN THE LAST YEAR	YES, DURING THE LAST YEAR

10. Has a relative or friend or a doctor or other health worker, been concerned about your drinking or suggested you cut down?

NO	YES, BUT NOT IN THE LAST YEAR	YES, DURING THE LAST YEAR

* One drink is (give national examples).

Fig. 10.3. World Health Organization 'core' screening instrument.

Item 1:			
	Never	-	0
	Monthly or less	-	1
	Two to four times a month	-	2
	Two to three times a week	-	3
	Four or more times a week	-	4
Item 2:			
	1–2 drinks	-	0
	3–4 drinks	-	1
	5–6 drinks	-	2
	7–9 drinks	-	3
	10+ drinks	-	4
Items 3–8:			
	Never	-	0
	Less than monthly	-	1
	Monthly	-	2
	Weekly	-	3
	Daily or almost daily	-	4
Items 9 & 10			
	No	-	0
	Yes, but not in the last year	-	2
	Yes, during the last year	-	4

The maximum possible score is 40.

Fig. 10.4. Scoring for the World Health Organization 'core' screening instrument.

in general practice (Wiseman *et al.* 1982) found that 3.5 per cent of patients aged over 15 years gave a positive result. Of the 35 patients with positive readings, 11 were not previously thought to have a problem related to alcohol. It is likely that a considerable number of heavy drinkers are missed by the alcohol meter because they have not actually been drinking shortly before the breath test. Alcohol meters therefore have limited usefulness in general practice.

Biological markers

The most commonly used biological markers of excessive alcohol consumption are mean cell volume (MCV) and gamma-glutamyl transpeptidase (gamma-GT) (Chick *et al.* 1981). Of these, gamma-GT is a better predictor than MCV. Although the MCV is related to alcohol consumption, a raised MCV is very unreliable as a screening test. The proportion of heavy drinkers who have an MCV over 98 fl ranges somewhere between 20 and 30 per cent and the false-positive rate is between four and six per cent.

There is a positive relationship between alcohol consumption and gamma-GT levels. Increased gamma-GT activity in the serum can be observed after a few weeks of alcohol intake. Following reduction in drinking, serum gamma-GT levels rapidly fall, returning to normal levels within two to four weeks. The rise of the enzyme in the serum is primarily due to hepatic enzyme induction. Nevertheless, gamma-GT is not very good as a screening instrument. The proportion of heavy drinkers with a raised level, more than 50 i.u./l, is about 50 per cent. The false-positive rate is between 10 to 20 per cent. Other causes of a raised gamma-GT include diseases of the liver, biliary tract, and pancreas. Normal values for gamma-GT are given in Chapter 11. The most important use of gamma-GT is for monitoring changes in alcohol consumption.

References

Chick, J., Kreightman, N., and Plant, M. (1981). Mean cell volume and gamma-glutamyl transpeptidase as markers of drinking in working men. *Lancet,* **1,** 1249–51.

Mayfield, D., McLeod, G., and Hall, P. (1974). The CAGE questionnaire: validation of a new alcoholism screening instrument. *American Journal of Psychiatry,* **131,** 1121–3.

Pokorny, A.D. *et al.* (1972). The brief MAST: a shortened version of the Michigan Alcoholism Screening Test. *American Journal of Psychiatry,* **129,** 342–5.

Saunders, J.B. and Aasland, O.G. (1987). *WHO collaborative project of identification and treatment of persons with harmful alcohol consumption.* Report on Phase 1: Development of a screening instrument. Geneva, WHO.

Saunders, W.M., and Kershaw, P.W. (1980). Screening tests for alcoholism—findings from a community study. *British Journal of Addiction,* **75,** 37–41.

Wiseman, S.M., Thompson, P.V., Barnett, J.M., Jenns, M., and Wilton, J. (1982). Use of an alcoholmeter to detect problem drinkers. *British Medical Journal*, **285,** 1089–90.

11 Management of different risk levels of alcohol consumption

Classification

Using information obtained about alcohol consumption, patients can be classified and put into one of three categories:

Classification	*Units consumed per week*	*Expected numbers (practice 2000)*
Low	Women less than 15	700
	Men less than 20	500
Intermediate	Women 15–35	75
	Men 20–50	150
High	Women more than 36	15
	Men more than 51	50

Vulnerability

Some people are particularly vulnerable to the effects of alcohol:

1. Children and the very old show increased susceptibility to the effects of alcohol.
2. Patients with chronic illness, e.g. diabetes, epilepsy, raised blood pressure, and some gastro-intestinal conditions.
3. Psychological conditions ranging from anxiety and depression to psychosis and brain damage.

4. Certain medications interact with alcohol (see Table 7.1).
5. Harmful life-styles including poor diet, obesity, and heavy smoking.
6. Unemployment.

Women are harmed at lower levels of consumption than men.

Each practice needs to develop its own plans for assessing and managing the problems which arise from the use of alcohol.

SUGGESTED MANAGEMENT PLAN

Low	Review 5 yearly (*Note*: pregnancy)
Intermediate Not vulnerable	Advise to reduce consumption Review yearly
Intermediate Vulnerable	Assess—advise to reduce Consumption review yearly
High	Assess—advise to reduce consumption—monitor closely

Low consumption—'normal vulnerability'

The large majority of any practice population will consist of people who drink less than 15 units (women) or 20 units (men) weekly and show no extra vulnerability as listed above. The general practitioner should record the current level of consumption, discuss any concerns about drinking which the patient may have, provide simple information such as the HEA booklet, *That's the limit* and arrange for review after, say, five years or whenever any significant change occurs in their life (e.g. pregnancy or bereavement).

Low consumption—'high vulnerability'

Some of those who have low consumption but high vulnerability will suffer from transient conditions, and alcohol should be kept on the agenda for any consultations for those conditions. Review should be arranged after, say, three years.

Intermediate consumption—'normal vulnerability'

Patients who normally drink between 15–35 units (women) and 20–50 units (men) a week should be given advice and information about the risks they are taking, encouragement and help in reducing consumption and offered review in, say, a year.

Intermediate consumption—'high vulnerability'

Those drinking the same amount but who are more vulnerable should be assessed for existing harms in social, psychological, and physical terms, advised about reducing consumption and supported in that endeavour whether by the doctor or another team member.

High consumption

Anyone consuming about 35 units (women) and 50 units (men) weekly will require fuller assessment, with advice, support, and regular follow-up.

References

That's the limit (1986) Health Education Authority, London.

12 Minimal intervention

The following intervention strategy is intended to be used primarily for *the prevention of alcohol problems. It is not intended for the management of patients who have already been severely damaged by alcohol.*

Who needs it

1. All men drinking at least 35 units a week.

2. All women drinking at least 21 units a week.

KEEP A TRACK OF WHAT YOU DRINK OVER THE NEXT TWO WEEKS

STARTING DATE

DAY	Beer, Cider (pints)	Spirits (measures)	Sherry, Wine etc.	Units
SUN				
MON				
TUE				
WED				
THU				
FRI				
SAT				
			WEEK'S TOTAL	

DAY	Beer, Cider (pints)	Spirits (measures)	Sherry, Wine etc.	Units
SUN				
MON				
TUE				
WED				
THU				
FRI				
SAT				
			WEEK'S TOTAL	

Fig. 12.1. A 'drinks' diary.

HOW MANY UNITS OF ALCOHOL IN YOUR DRINK?

		UNITS OF ALCOHOL
BEERS AND LAGERS		
Ordinary strengh beer or lager	½ pint	1
	1 pint	2
	1 can	1½
Export beer	1 pint	2½
	1 can	2
Strong ale or lager	½ pint	2
	1 pint	4
	1 can	3
Extra strength beer or lager	½ pint	2½
	1 pint	5
	1 can	2
CIDERS		
Average cider	½ pint	1½
	1 pint	3
	quart bottle	6
Strong cider	½ pint	2
	1 pint	4
	quart bottle	8
SPIRITS		
	1 standard single measure	1
	1 bottle	30
TABLE WINE		
(including cider wine and barley wine)	1 standard glass	1
	1 bottle	7
	1 litre bottle	10
SHERRY AND FORTIFIED WINE		
	1 standard small measure	1
	1 bottle	12

1 UNIT ALCOHOL = 1 STANDARD DRINK

Fig. 12.2. Conversion chart.

Men drinking between 20–35 units a week should be kept under careful review as should women drinking between 14–21 units per week.

Note:
In the case of people aged under 18 or over 64, lower levels may be appropriate. For pregnant women much lower levels may be appropriate because of risk to the baby (e.g. 1 or 2 units once or twice a week).

It is acceptable for practice staff, of course, to decide on different limits for specific patients.

Components

1. Ask the patient if they believe that their alcohol is affecting their health and/or life.

2. Make a note of the patient's drinking habits: weekly consumption/types of drink/regular heavy drinking days, etc.

3. Fill in a drinks diary recording consumption for the previous seven days. Start with the previous day and work backwards. Recall is assisted by asking about morning, lunch-time, and evening of each day (Figs. 12.1–12.2)

4. Indicate the patient's position on the histogram (Fig. 12.3). This will correct beliefs about 'normality' of the patient's own consumption or that of his peers.

5. Mention the risks of increased drinking, such as:

   Accidents and injuries
   Weight problems
   Stomach upsets
   Liver disease
   Headaches
   Anxiety and depression
   Sexual difficulties
   Difficulties in sleeping
   Raised blood pressure
   Hangover

6. Mention the benefits of reduced drinking, such as:

   Financial savings
   Safer driving
   Improved concentration at work
   Improved general health

   Plus any factors specific to the individual patient.

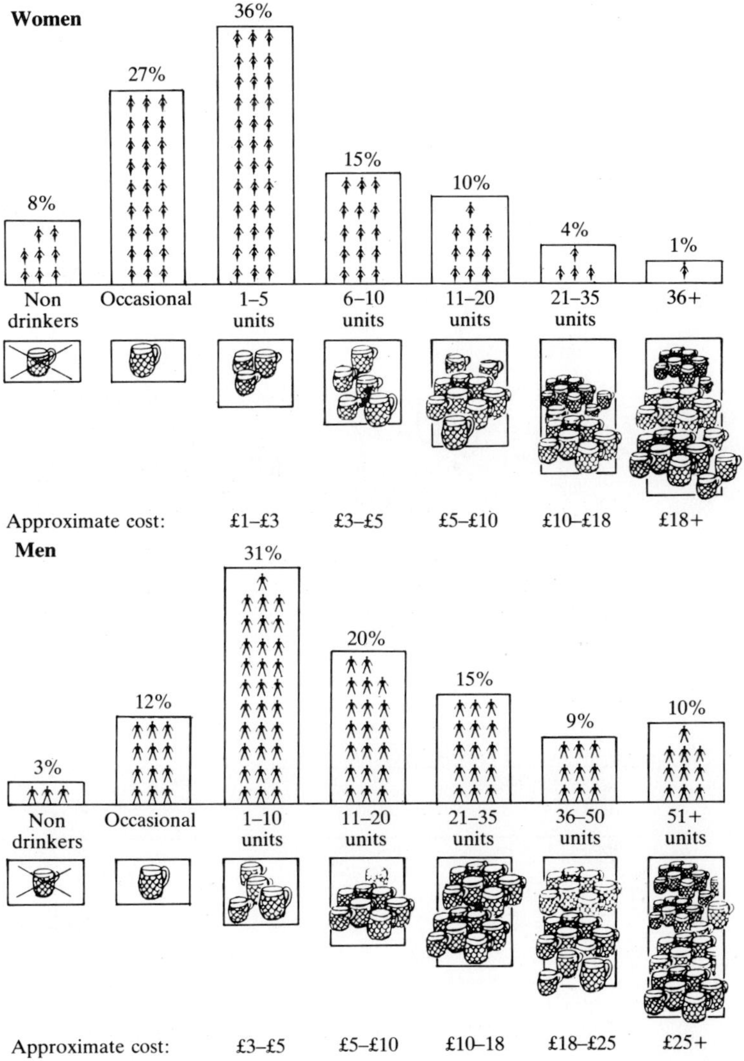

Fig. 12.3. Units of alcohol consumed per week in England and Wales. From Wallace and Haines. Revised by Anderson and Jones Alcohol Project (1987).

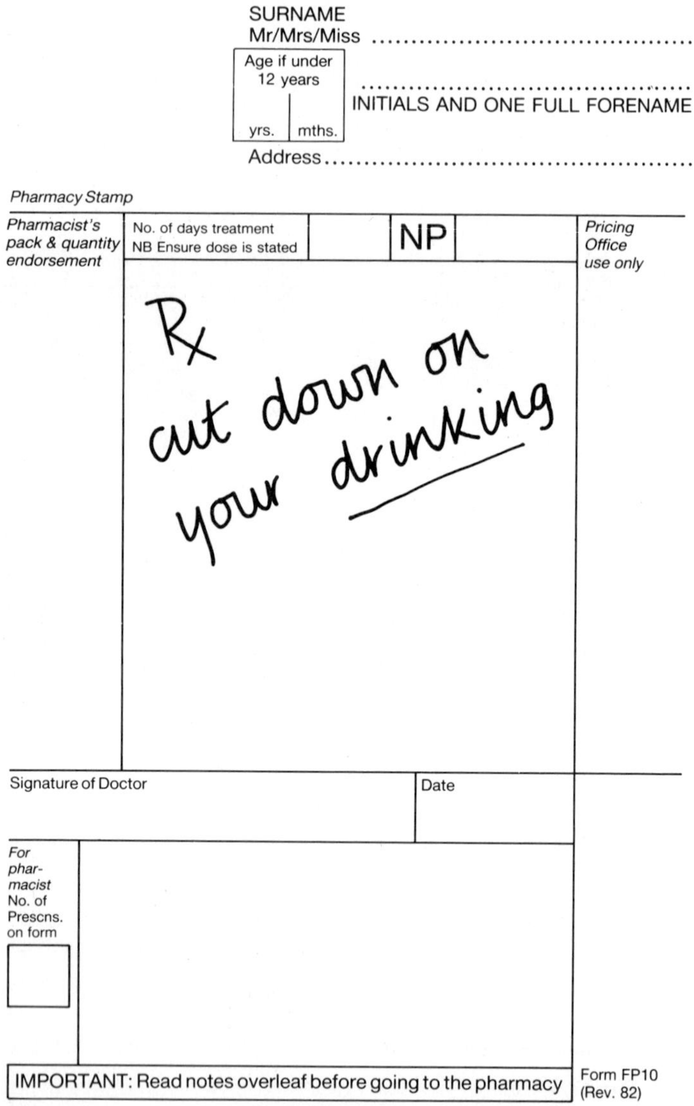

SURNAME
Mr/Mrs/Miss ....

Age if under 12 years

yrs. | mths.

....
INITIALS AND ONE FULL FORENAME

Address..

Pharmacy Stamp

Pharmacist's pack & quantity endorsement

No. of days treatment
NB Ensure dose is stated

NP

Pricing Office use only

Rx
cut down on
your drinking

Signature of Doctor

Date

For phar-macist
No. of Prescns. on form

IMPORTANT: Read notes overleaf before going to the pharmacy

Form FP10
(Rev. 82)

Fig. 12.4. *Cut down on your drinking* booklet (available from Health Education Authority).

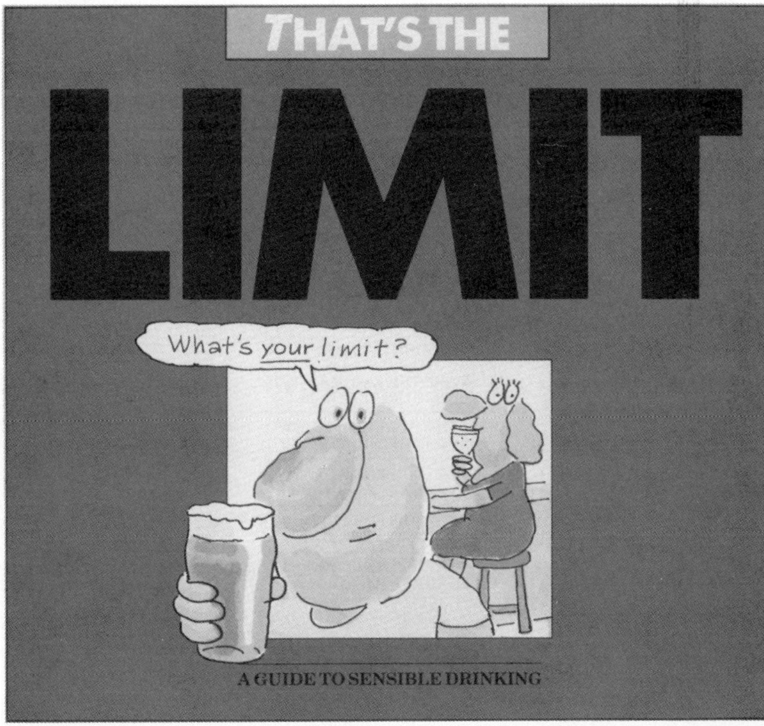

Fig. 12.5. *That's the limit* booklet (available from Health Education Authority).

7. Give firm but friendly advice to cut down. Bearing in mind individual circumstances in general, it is suggested that:
   You advise men:
   NOT to drink more than 20 units per week
   You advise women:
   NOT to drink more than 15 units per week

8. Give the patient literature such as the *cut down on your drinking* booklet or *That's the limit* (Figs 12.4 and 12.5).

9. Arrange a follow-up appointment within the following two to four weeks. Explain that you will be asking about the patient's alcohol consumption at future attendance at surgery.

Recording keeping

Note the interview and the date in the patient's notes. You may also wish to attach a sticker inside or outside the notes to remind you to check the patient's consumption at their next consultation.

References

Cut down on your drinking pack (1987). Health Education Authority and Alcohol Concern, London.
That's the limit (1986). Health Education Authority, London.

13 Assessment of alcohol consumption

Chapters 9 and 11 discussed the *measurement* of patients' alcohol consumption and the appropriate *management* response to various risk levels based on the information obtained. Chapter 12 described a brief intervention for those in the upper end of the moderate risk category. A minority of patients will require a little extra time and attention and this chapter describes this *fuller assessment*.

Who needs to be assessed?

1. All those patients whose drinking identifies them as in the *heavy* category.

2. All those in the *moderate* drinking category who are vulnerable in relation to associated risks factors (Chapter 11).
3. Patients who record a high positive profile on the following check-list:

Alcohol problems check-list

Health problems

Stomach upsets?
Sickness, vomiting?
Difficulty sleeping?
Easily upset?
Depressed?
Indigestion?
Diarrhoea, loose bowels?
Tiredness or difficulty concentrating?
Anxiety symptoms?
Panic attacks?

Social problems
Arguments at home about drinking?
Arguments at home made worse by drinking?
Family member threated to leave because of drinking?
Been asked to leave pub/party, etc. because drunk?
Money worries because of drinking?
Problems with police because of drinking?

Accidents/work problems
Trouble at work because of drinking?
Absence from work because of drinking?
Been in accident because of drinking?

Symptoms of developing tolerance
Unable to keep to a drink limit?
Difficulty preventing getting drunk?
Restless without a drink?
Trembling after drinking the day before?
Drinking in the morning?

How to assess

Full assessment may take some time. It is sometimes helpful to divide it between surgeries.

History taking

Together with the patient, complete a seven-day drink diary for the week prior to consultation. You can help in the recall by working backwards one day at a time and asking about the day in components; e.g. morning/lunch-time/evening.

As always in medical assessment the past history is vital. It is essential to discover:

When heavy drinking started.
Events which were linked at the time.
Accounts of any bouts of heavier drinking including the days before and after, what the patient felt and thought at the time.
Information about previous attempts to cut down or abstain.
The events surrounding relapses.
Attitudes and behaviour of those close to the patient.
A brief summary of early life and upbringing.

Examination

General practitioners are expert at physical assessment in the surgery. As a minimum, a check should be made on: pulse and blood pressure; liver for tenderness or enlargement; hands for tremor or sweating; breath for smell of alcohol; height and weight.

Investigations

The following two tests should be undertaken:
MCV and gamma-glutamyl transaminase.

Normal range of values for laboratory tests

MCV	78–98 g/dl
γ-GT	Male less than 28 i.u./l
	Female less than 18 i.u./l

In making an assessment the primary objective should be to obtain and share information and understanding with the patient so that decisions can be made about management. Ideally, the patient should clarify the issues around his drinking and reach decisions on his own without explicit advice being offered. This is a key to effective counselling and it represents a shift of approach for doctors and other medical staff who are traditionally seen as dispensers of advice. The desired goal of intervention is for the patient to offer strategies for change which are then more likely to be met.

Some patients, probably a minority, may be unwilling or unable to be honest with their doctor and/or themselves. The responses should be to discontinue direct questioning and explore the issues around the denial or blocking. If the reluctance persists record the interview in the notes and mark for interview on another occasion.

14 Intervention with high-risk patients

This more intensive intervention will only be necessary for a small minority of patients drinking heavily (at least 35 units for women and 50 for men).

Reducing consumption

The aim of responding to a patient who is drinking heavily or has problems related to alcohol is:

To reduce consumption
To help with the harms that alcohol is causing

People may be at one of three stages of belief about their drinking: (1) pre-understanding; (2) understanding; (3) action (Prochaska and Diclemente 1985).

Pre-understanding

At this stage the person has not thought about harmful drinking and needs help in understanding the relationship between consumption and harm.

Understanding

At this stage the patient has thought about his or her drinking but has not done anything about it. The patient needs help in decision-making, weighing-up, and altering the balance sheet of the good and harmful effects of drinking.

Action

When this stage is reached the person is actually trying to do something about reducing consumption and may need some help.

The aim of intervention with high-risk patients is to help the patient progress through these key stages.

Moving from understanding to action

Chapter 12 discusses the use of a *drinks diary* for an accurate calculation in units of the patient's consumption. This in itself may be an important part of therapy and many people are surprised to find out how much alcohol they are actually consuming a week.

The information from the diary can be discussed with the patient and realistic goals for reduction reached by mutual agreement. List the problems related to alcohol experienced by the patient. For the first time he or she may learn how some symptoms are related to alcohol and thus accept the need for change.

It is effective to relate the patients' presenting symptoms to their alcohol consumption where appropriate.

Explain the chemical, and pharmacological effects of alcohol and about the ways in which tolerance develops and the nature of early withdrawal symptoms.

The patient should be told the results of blood tests.

Even if the patient understands the harm his drinking is causing he may decide *against* taking immediate steps to cut down. In this case he can be given information in case he changes his mind and he can be told that the issue will be discussed in future consultations.

Note: Record the interview in notes and tag for reminder.

Some people will respond quickly to the strategies outlined above. Others may need further help and the same process must be repeated as often as necessary in spite of past failures.

The effort the individual is making must be positively reinforced by the general practitioner/nurse. Censure, disapproval, and guilt-inducing responses from those working with patients struggling to reduce consumption is never productive for effective behavioural change. Conversely, approval and encouragement can be highly motivating rewards.

Goals for change

Discover from the patient what he or she wants and reach an agreement or contract on goals for change.

Long-term goals will depend on previous history.

If the drinking is excessive although hitherto harm free, advice can be given about sensible levels of drinking.

Other drinkers with established problems should also aim to drink less.

For some, abstinence remains the preferable goal. This group includes those who demonstrate severe withdrawal symptoms from alcohol, have severe physical damage or who have systematically tried controlled drinking without success (Heather and Robertson 1983).

How to change

The main aim of therapy is to reduce alcohol consumption. The way to do this is to encourage self-management and education—the first step being to start self-monitoring (Kanfer and Brusemeyer 1982; Kanfer and Grimm 1980).

The drinks diary

This involves keeping a diary of *how much* is drunk . . . *when, where*, and *with whom*.

Show the patient how to record drinking and convert the amount of alcohol consumed into units.

The diary should be completed each day and kept for a few weeks. It should be referred to at consultations and progress discussed. Note from the diary when the patient drank more than intended or when drinking has caused trouble. This may have been associated with:

Times of the day or certain days of the week.
People with whom drinking occurs.
Whether the patient was hungry or thirsty.
How the patient was feeling emotionally—anxious, under stress, frustrated, angry, depressed.
Conflicts with other people or rows within the family.

The patient should be helped to:

Anticipate these circumstances.
Avoid 'dangerous' circumstances.
Cope with them in alternative ways.

For example, he may have become used to a drink at a certain time, on the way home from work and so acquired a strong urge to drink then.

He should avoid the situation and confine his drinking to safe occasions where he has drunk sensibly in the past.

Useful tips

It is also useful to give advice on how to consume less alcohol. Some useful tips are to:

Take non-alcoholic drinks
Take smaller sips
Sip less often and take small sips. Count the number of sips it takes to

finish a glass, and then try increasing the number for the next glass and so on.

Occupy yourself

Do something else enjoyable while drinking that will help distract attention from the glass, and drink more slowly. For example, eating, listening to music, darts, talking, and so on.

Change the drink

Changing the type of drink can help break old habits and reduce the amount drunk.

Drink for the taste

Drink more slowly and enjoy the flavour.

Imitate the slow drinker

Identify someone who drinks slowly and become a shadow, not picking up the glass until he does.

Put the glass down between sips

If the glass is held it will be drunk more often. Do something else with your hands instead of lifting the glass to the lips.

Dilute spirits

Top up spirits with non-alcoholic mixers.

Reduce amounts in rounds

Buy your own drinks or one round and then go solo; do not buy yourself a drink when it is your round; order non-alcoholic drinks every so often.

Drink and eat

Eat before drinking or whilst drinking; this slows down the absorption of alcohol and doing something else may also reduce the amount drunk.

Take days of rest

Abstain from alcohol at least one day per week, or preferably two, three, or even four days per week. Take up other forms of entertainment or relaxation.

Start later

Start drinking later than usual; for example, go to the pub later.

Learn to refuse drinks

Consider ways of refusing drinks, for example: 'No thanks, I'm cutting down', or 'Not tonight, I've got a bad stomach'.

Maintaining reduced drinking

1. It is essential to offer follow-up when progress can be reviewed, continuing help and support offered, as well as further advice on managing difficulties.
2. The drinks' diary should be reviewed.
3. Progress should be reviewed regularly over a year. The first six months often give a good impression of longer-term prognosis; see Fig. 14.1.
4. Blood tests are a useful means of monitoring progress. The results and implications can be discussed with the patient. (γg-GT returns rapidly to normal with abstention and may return to normal if measured 48 hours after the last drink.)

Preventing relapse

Many people will experience some form of relapse and will need to be warned about this. Both doctor and patient need to be aware of

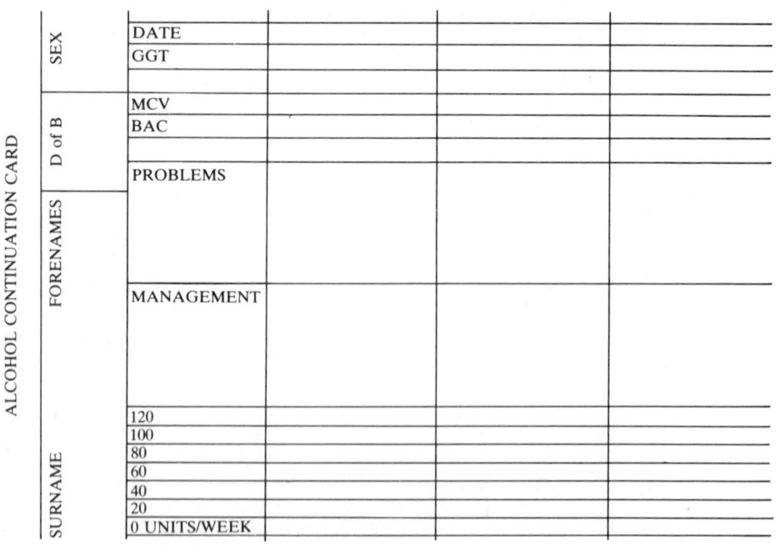

Fig. 14.1. Alcohol continuation card.

the sort of problems which are likely to cause a relapse and it is useful to draw up a list or inventory of relapse precipitants. They can then plan systematic strategies to avoid relapse either by using alternative coping methods or by making substantial changes in life-style (Marlatt and George 1984).

Relapse should not be regarded as a loss of all that has been achieved but as an opportunity for the patient to learn more about himself and his problem. Once the relapse has been openly discussed the patient can recognize strategies for preventing a further recurrence.

Psychological therapies

To help maintain reduced drinking there may be a need for specific behavioural therapies. Discussions about management will depend on the reasons for the drinking. Relaxation training for those individuals who drink in response to stress is helpful; alternatives may be yoga or meditation. Those who are isolated or find it difficult to make friends may benefit from social skills training. There may be a need for marital or family therapy as family, marital or sexual discord may have preceded the drinking or have resulted from it. Finally, help may be needed in connection with work, as there are links between certain occupations and heavy drinking (see Table 3.1).

Working with the family

Many studies have stressed the importance of family support (Harwin 1982), and Saunders and Kershaw (1979) confirmed this when they studied people who considered that they had had a drinking problem in the past but no longer. When these people were asked for reasons, by far the most common was 'marriage'. Obtaining work, or improvements in work conditions were among others.

Partners of excessive drinkers usually suffer greatly—psychologically, physically, and socially.

It is important to listen and understand before attempting to help, and not to blame either partner for the occurrence of the problems.

Both partners should be encouraged to accept responsibility for their own behaviour and thus their own symptoms and feelings, and be helped to make whatever changes seem desirable for their own good and that of their partner.

Very often the partner has been behaving in such a way that the drinker has actively been prevented from seeing that the drink is causing problems; for example, he or she may have covered up by giving excuses for the drinker avoiding work, or by paying his debts. Many therefore need counselling to help them cope with these feelings and to avoid drink-sustaining behaviour within the family. It may be only when the partner ceases this cover-up that the drinker can face the reality of his situation.

The partner may be encouraged to follow the same lines, for example, by altering the balance sheet in favour of reduced drinking. He or she should reward non-drinking times, and be careful not to 'reward' drinking times by giving in as an 'easy option' when faced with an acute problem. Rewards are a valuable way of helping the drinker shift his position. It is important, therefore, for the partner to recognize the times when drinking behaviour has been rewarded and sober behaviour punished.

Referral sources

The majority of heavy drinkers and patients with alcohol problems can be helped by support from members of the primary care team and their own families.

However, there are some whose problems are more severe or who lack a supportive environment who may need referring on to a specialist agency.

When a referral is made *it is important nonetheless to maintain your relationship with the patient* and give a further appointment to discuss what took place.

Without this continuing contact, the referral may feel like a rejection.

Many areas have local councils on alcohol, voluntary agencies whose responsibilities include co-ordinating available services and which provide counselling and advice for heavy drinkers and their families. Addresses of local councils may be found in the telephone directory, or alternatively Alcohol Concern (see p. 84) publishes a directory of national and local services.

Community alcohol teams (CATs) are multidisciplinary groups, often involving social workers, probation officers, psychiatric nurses, counsellors, psychologists, and others, which are often attached to, or at least have close links with, alcohol treatment units.

Alcoholics Anonymous provides a supportive self-help group. It asks members to acknowledge that they are 'alcoholic' and that abstinence is the only way to recovery. Al-Anon and Al-Teen provide support for the spouses and teenage children of problem drinkers. Addresses are in the telephone directory.

Alcohol treatment units are usually associated with psychiatric units, have facilities for detoxification and offer a range of approaches to treatment.

References

Harwin, J. (1982). The excessive drinker and the family: Approaches to treatment. In *Alcohol and the family* (ed. J. Orford and J. Harwin), Croom Helm, London.

Heather, N. and Robertson, I. (1983). *Controlled drinking*. Methuen, London.

Kanfer, F.H. and Brusemeyer, J.R. (1982). The use of problem solving and decision making in behaviour therapy. *Clinical Psychology Review*, **2,** 239–66.

Kanfer, F.H. and Grimm, L.G. (1980). Managing clinical change. A process model of therapy. *Behaviour Modification*, **4,** 419–44.

Marlatt, G.A. and George, W.H. (1984). Relapse prevention: Introduction and overview of the model. *British Journal of Addiction*, **79,** 261–73.

Prochaska, J.O. and Diclemente, C.C. (1985). *The transtheoretical approach: Crossing traditional boundaries of therapy*. Illinois, Dow Jones-Irwin.

Saunders, W. and Kershaw, P. (1979). Spontaneous remission from alcoholism—a community study. *British Journal of Addiction*, **74,** 251–66.

15 Detoxification

Who needs it?

1. A tiny minority of patients who give a history of severe withdrawal symptoms, and/or
2. show signs of withdrawal at consultation.

Where can detoxification be carried out?

1. At home (provided that family support is available).
2. In a general hospital.
3. In an alcoholic treatment unit.

Most detoxification can safely take place at home.

The process of detoxification is important in establishing the doctor/patient relationship.

The patient will be highly dependent on good medical care and may feel vulnerable and *it is important for the patient to be seen daily during this phase by his doctor, practice nurse, community psychiatric nurse or other member of the practice team to monitor the detoxification and foster the relationship.*

It is also a valuable time for assessment of the patient and the rest of the family.

Detoxification drugs

Diazepam is the preferred drug. The starting dose and its duration is determined by the anticipated severity of withdrawal based on previous withdrawal history.

The present pattern is likely to repeat that of previous withdrawals unless the previous drinking has been different. It is also important to ensure that the patient has not been using or abusing other drugs, because tolerance to Diazepam may have developed which would require a longer regime at larger doses.

Dosage

For withdrawals at home which are expected to be severe, a maximum of 20 mg of Diazepam, four times a day, *reducing daily and ending after seven days may be necessary*; in most cases much less (usually 5 mg) is indicated.

The medication should be supervised closely and not supplied in large quantities at a time.

Note: If the patient gives a history of severe delirium tremens and/or withdrawal fits, or if his social circumstances are such that proper care is not available at home, then admission to hospital has to be considered.

Vitamins

Vitamins should be given during detoxification. Parentrovite, one pair of high potency ampoules, a dose of which, given intramuscularly or intravenously daily for five days is suggested, followed by oral medication.

Because hypoglycaemia can sometimes occur, sugary fluids should always be encouraged.

Family support

Advising the family and the patient on the symptoms, signs, duration, and management of detoxification helps to ensure a safe and constructive withdrawal.

16 The effectiveness of intervention

There is good evidence that heavy drinkers want to cut down on their drinking and that when treatment is available they come forward for help (Plant *et al.* 1979; Cust 1980).

There is also good evidence to suggest that general practitioners should be able to do a great deal to help patients who are drinking heavily (Orford and Edwards 1977; Heather 1985; Wallace *et al.* in press).

Evidence about smoking

The effectiveness of general practitioners' advice to their patients to stop smoking was shown in the study by Jamrozik *et al.* (1984) (Fig. 16.1).

The results indicated that general practitioners who adopted a simple protocol of advice and follow-up could expect about 25 long-term successes per annum. If all general practitioners in the UK participated, the total number of ex-smokers per year would exceed half a million.

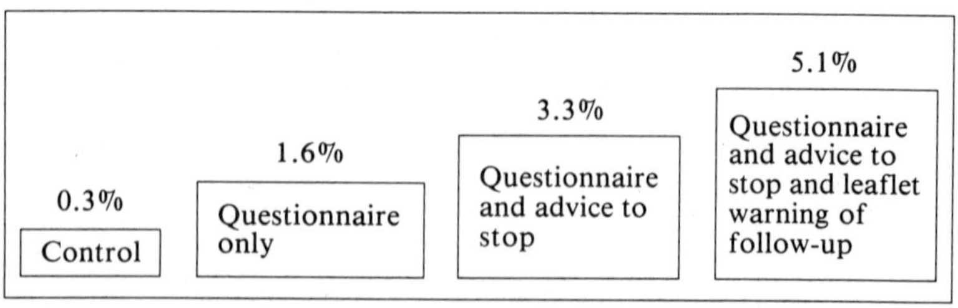

Fig. 16.1. Percentage of smokers who had stopped smoking at the end of a year, 1984.

Evidence about drinking

The DRAMS scheme

A study by Heather *et al.* (1987) using the DRAMS scheme (Drinking Reasonably And Moderately with Self-control) which is a minimal intervention method demonstrated that at six months follow-up general practitioners' advice was effective in reducing the alcohol consumption of heavy drinkers (Fig. 16.2).

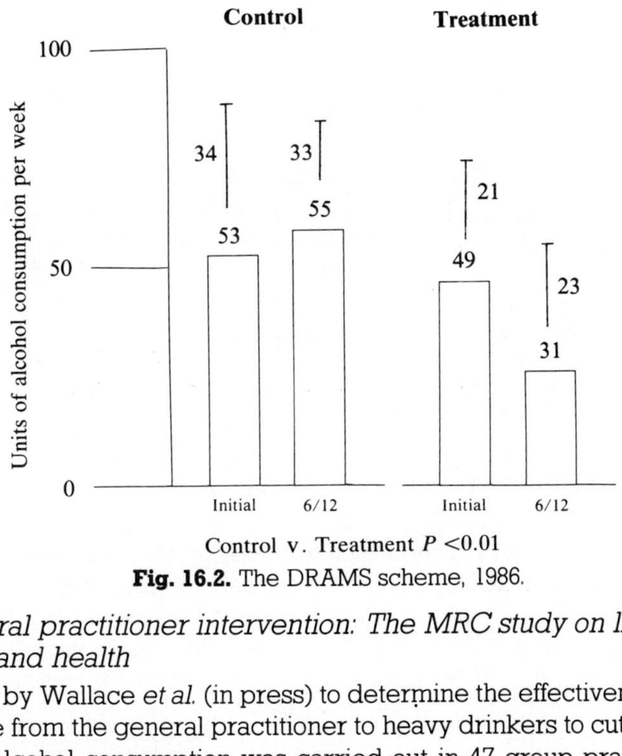

Fig. 16.2. The DRAMS scheme, 1986.

General practitioner intervention: The MRC study on life-style and health

A trial by Wallace *et al.* (in press) to determine the effectiveness of advice from the general practitioner to heavy drinkers to cut down their alcohol consumption was carried out in 47 group practices. Initial screening using the Health Survey Questionnaire in 62 153 patients aged 17–69 followed by an interview resulted in 917 heavy drinkers (men drinking at least 35 units a week and women drinking 21 units or more) being randomized to either treatment or control groups. Patients in the treatment group were interviewed by their general practitioner, received advice and information about how to reduce their consumption, and follow-up within one month and again at four, seven, and 10 months.

At one year, a mean reduction in consumption of 18.2 units/week had occurred in the treated men compared with a reduction of 8.1 units/week in controls. The proportion of men with excessive consumption at interview had dropped by 43.7 per cent in the treatment group compared with 25.5 per cent in the control group. A mean reduction in weekly consumption of 11.5 units occurred in treated women compared with 6.3 units in controls and the proportionate reduction of excessive drinkers in treatment and control groups was 47.7 and 29.2 per cent respectively. The mean value of gamma-glutamyl transpeptidase dropped significantly more in the treated men (−2.37 i.u./l) than in the controls (+1.12 i.u./l) at one year, and the reduction in both consumption and gamma-glutamyl transpeptidase increased with the number of general practitioner interventions.

On the basis of the results, the authors calculated that advice from general practitioners in the UK could result, each year, in a reduction to moderate levels the alcohol consumption of some 210 000 men and 135 000 women who currently drink to excess.

Counselling heavy drinkers on medical wards (Chick *et al.* 1985)

A total of 731 men admitted to hospital wards were interviewed to identify heavy drinkers who had not received previous treatment and who had some social support: 156 were allocated to one of two groups. One group received a 20 minute session of counselling about their drinking habits from a nurse. The other group received only routine medical care. After one year, 124 patients were re-interviewed. The patients given counselling showed significant improvements compared with the controls:

Patients given	*Improved*	*Not improved*
Counselling (n=78)	34	31
Controls (n=78)	20	39

Identification and intervention of heavy drinking in middle-aged men, Malmo, Sweden (Kristenson *et al.* 1982)

The study sample consisted of 585 men (born 1926–33) randomly allocated to either an intervention group or a control group. Two and four years after screening, the gamma-glutamyl transpeptidase values in both groups were significantly decreased. There were differences, however, between the two groups with regard to sick absenteeism, hospitalisation, and mortality. Compared with the control group a significant reduction was found in the treatment group:

In sick absence by 80 per cent at 4-year follow-up.
In hospital days by 60 per cent at 5-year follow-up.
In mortality by 50 per cent at 6-year follow-up.

The intervention programme, which included repeated encouragement to lower overall alcohol consumption and bio-feedback information in the form of gamma-glutamyl transpeptidase measurements was effective in preventing medico-social consequences of heavy drinking.

References

Chick, J., Lloyd, G., and Crombie, E. (1985). Counselling problem drinkers in medical wards. *British Medical Journal*, **290,** 965–7.

Cust, G. (1980). Health education about alcohol in the Tyne tees area. In *Aspects of alcohol and drug dependence.* (eds. Madden, J.S., Walker, R., and Kenyor, W.H.), 117–22, Pitman Medical, Bath.

Heather, N. (1985). Minimal treatment interventions for problem drinkers. In *Current issues in clinical psychology* (ed. G. Edwards, and M. Gill), Vol. 4, Plenum, London.

Heather, N., Campion, P.D., Neville, R.G., and MacCabe, D. (1987). Evaluation of a controlled drinking minimal intervention (the DRAMS scheme) in general practice. *Journal of the Royal College of General Practitioners*, **37,** 358–63.

Jamrozik, K. *et al.* (1984). Controlled trial of three different anti-smoking interventions in general practice. *British Medical Journal*, **288,** 1499–503.

Kristenson, H. *et al.* (1983). Identification and intervention of heavy drinking in middle-aged men; results and follow-up of 24–60 months of long-term study with randomised controls. *Alcoholism, Clinical and Experimental Research,* **7,** 203–9.

Orford, J. and Edwards, G. (1977). *Alcoholism: A comparison of treatment and advice with a study of the influence of marriage.* Oxford University Press.

Plant, M.A., Piries, F., and Kreitman, N. (1979). Evaluation of the Scottish Health Education Unit's 1976 campaign on alcoholism. *Social Psychiatry,* **14,** 11–24.

Wallace, P.G., Cutler, S., and Haines, A.P. Randomised controlled trial of general practitioner intervention in patients with excessive alcohol consumption: findings of the MRC's general practice research framework study on lifestyle and health. *British Medical Journal.* (In press).

17 Audit and research

Information and assessment

General practices could find out the numbers of patients/proportions of different groups in which there is evidence that:

Alcohol has been asked about.
Alcohol consumption has been recorded.
Harm from alcohol has been assessed.
Counselling or further examination has been advised or performed.
Other family members have been involved.
The health of other family members has been checked.

This type of audt could examine the present state of affairs, and how that state has changed over the past years, and how it is affected by changes in practice policies.

Practice behaviour

Practices could examine the effects of introducing different systems of management including:

A morbidity index.
Use of leaflets and pamphlets.
Structured problems cards and flow cards.
Questionnaires offered by receptionists.
Postal questionnaires.
Computer questioning.

Practices could study the way in which policies were formulated and applied; the effect of involving the whole team in learning, assessing, and management; and the effect of asking practice members to review their own drinking habits.

The practice might also consider ways of working with local professionals, psychologists, and community alcohol teams, for example, and of extending these links to issues of prevention and health education, working with local magistrates, etc.

Outcome and results

Any practice will have numerous different management patterns, both selected and occurring spontaneously. Record systems could be planned to accommodate research into possible different outcomes: intervention; interviewing and counselling of different types; interventions involving families; different kinds of referral.

These outcomes can be assessed in terms of general health (questionnaire, consultations), health of families, future drinking patterns. The success of the practice could be measured in terms of work done, proportion of problems actively managed, job satisfaction, practicability of policies adopted, co-operative research with national and local bodies.

18 Local responses

Provision of information

Many local authorities, institutions, and individuals whose work has some reference to alcohol problems need regular information on the size and nature of alcohol problems in their community.

Media

The media is an important target group for information relating to prevention and excessive consumption:

(1) People who work in the media are amongst the highest consumers of alcohol, and
(2) they have a public responsibility to provide a balanced perspective of matters of public and social significance.

Some general practitioners are radio doctors or newspaper columnists and have opportunities to present the public health aspects of alcohol use. They should be at the front of informed contribution to the general debate, for example, at times of changes in the national budget.

Advertising

If alcohol advertisements appear to be in breach of the IBA and BCAP codes (see Chapter 19) *doctors should complain.* Unsatisfactory advertising practice could be changed.

At local level two initiatives might be developed:

1. Action can be taken to control poster advertising; in most areas the majority of poster sites are owned by the local authorities. They are in a position to control a highly usable form of mass communication.

Note: The voluntary code for cigarette advertising forbids any posters near schools.

2. The sponsorship of sport by tobacco companies is regulated by a code of practice which does not extend to alcohol. Opportunities exist at local level for registering concern at the involvement of alcohol companies in sports sponsorship.

Licensing

Many local individuals and organizations have a legitimate interest in licensing decisions and could be involved through, for example, a local licensing forum. Discussion might focus on the kinds of data which should be available when discussing general issues of need and specific problems, e.g. licensed premises and public disorder; the introduction, implementation, and support for an overall licensing strategy.

A major task of such a licensing forum would be to make representations to the licensing magistrates concerning the public health aspects of the availability of alcohol.

General practitioners are in an ideal position to set up and influence a licensing forum within their own locality.

Patient participation

As in all areas of health care it is important to involve the practice population and the local community. This will help the work of general practice and can be achieved through patient participation and other local community groups which could lead to the production of a practice report including information about the influences on alcohol consumption and alcohol-related harm in that community.

19 Prevention responses at national level

How could a general reduction in alcohol consumption be achieved?

There are four main areas in which a response to alcohol problems could be considered:

1. Price and fiscal policy.
2. Licensing laws.
3. Advertising.
4. Health education.

Price and fiscal policy

There is an inverse relationship between the real price of alcoholic beverages and the level of consumption per head and most indices of alcohol related harm (Figs 1.2 and 1.3, Chapter 1).

As the relative price of alcohol has fallen by over 50 per cent in the last 30 years alcohol consumption has increased accordingly (Fig. 19.1).

It has been suggested that high alcohol taxes may discriminate unfairly by leading to an uneven distribution of income after tax. In so far as the poor spend a higher proportion of their income on alcohol, they also pay a disproportionate share of the tax on alcohol. However, there are differences in the patterns of consumption of different types of alcoholic beverages which should be taken into account when making considerations of this kind. In Britain, beer appears more predominantly in the budgets of lower income groups, whereas higher income groups spend relatively more on spirits and wine.

The freedom of the British Government to fix taxation levels for alcoholic drinks is circumscribed by the Treaty of Rome. The

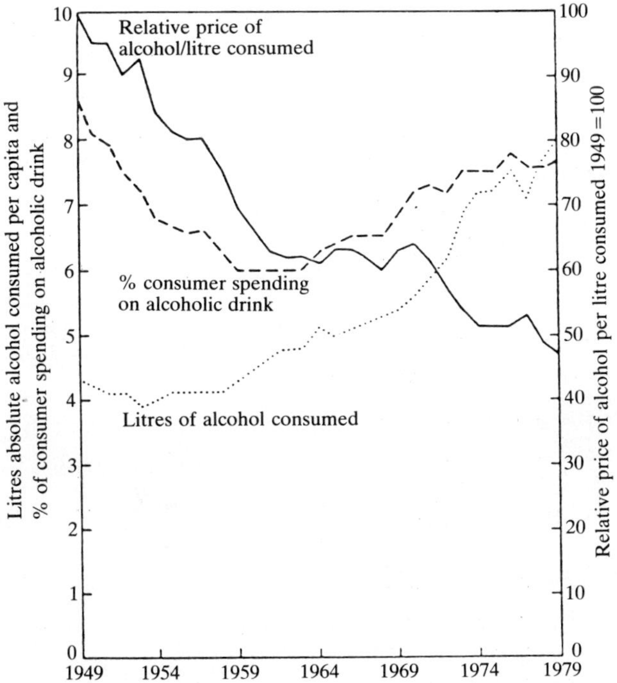

Fig. 19.1. The price relative to income per litre of absolute alcohol consumed in the UK, and the percentage of consumer spending on alcohol and litres of alcohol consumed, 1949–79.

European Community is seeking to create a common market in alcoholic drinks by removing internal barriers to trade. It is seeking to co-ordinate tax levels so that products are treated equally by the tax systems of the 10 member countries. If this were put into effect, it is estimated that alcohol consumption in this country would increase by 33 per cent for spirits and wine, and 10 per cent for beer.

Licensing laws

Licensing laws determine the terms and conditions under which alcohol can be made available to the public.

Although the issuing of licenses is a local matter, the licensing laws provide a legal framework within which the licensing magistrate must work.

The UK is near the bottom of international tables of alcohol consumption/related harm. In the past, our licensing laws contributed to this situation (Davies and Walsh 1983); (Fig. 19.2). The new licensing bill allows for public houses to open for 12 hours a day from Monday to Saturday in England and Wales.

Licensing laws were changed in Scotland in 1977–78. Contrary to popular belief, *alcohol consumption increased* as a result of the change—by 13 per cent between 1976 and 1984, and would have gone up even more but for rising unemployment (Goddard 1986).

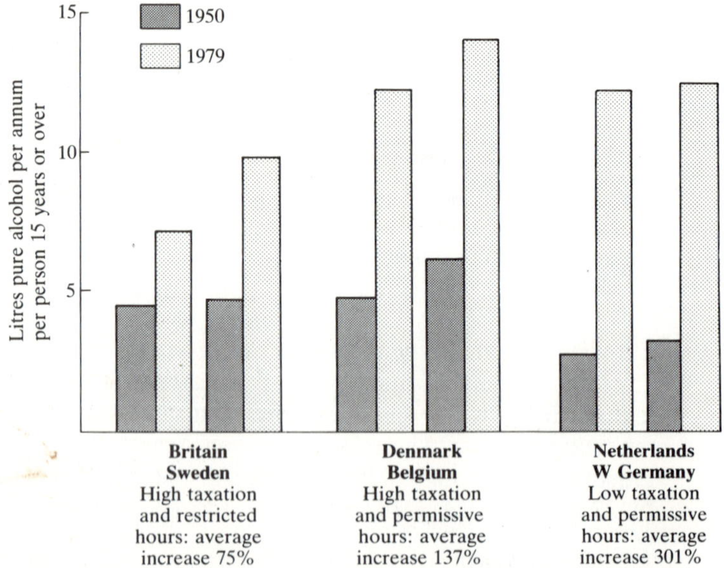

Fig. 19.2. Alcohol consumption trends in the six main beer-drinking countries in north-western Europe, 1950–79. From Davies and Walsh (1983).

Advertising

The alcohol industries claim that advertising affects brand choice rather than level of consumption.

However, there is evidence to show that changes in preferences tend to be additions rather than substitutions.

Brand or beverage switching may thus result in increased total alcohol consumption (Van Iwaarden 1983).

At least £200 million is spent annually on alcohol advertising and sponsorship.

Only £217 553 was spent on alcohol/health promotion by the Health Education Council for 1984/85.

It is widely agreed that the content of advertising material is important. The young and vulnerable may absorb harmful messages which will promote or reinforce harmful patterns of consumption. Controls of advertising content have been developed and alcohol advertising is specifically monitored by:

1. The Independent Broadcasting Authority (IBA) Code of Advertising Standards and Practice, 70 Brompton Road, London SW3 1EY.
2. Advertising Standards Authority (ASA) British Code of Advertising Practice (BCAP), Brook House, 2–16 Torrington Place, London WC1E 7HN.

Health education

The mass media exercise influence in a seductive and compelling way—alcohol health education should be no exception. However, health education about alcohol problems has not succeeded in reducing the problems, so far. A campaign in north-east England showed that specific media campaigns in alcohol education are very expensive and only modestly successful in imparting knowledge (Thorley 1985).

The mass media should be encouraged rather to put the prevention of alcohol-related problems onto their agenda and to get accurate information to the public.

The policy participants

The drinks trade

The drinks trade is immense, rich, and powerful.

–Six brewing groups control 80 per cent of the UK market and own about half of all public houses in the UK.
–40 per cent of wine distribution is controlled by eight companies. The largest distillers owned 45 malt distilleries and five grain distilleries in 1980.
–The links between production and distribution is extensive. Expansion has been rapid. By the 1970s it was estimated that the industry was employing 750 000 people.
–Production of alcoholic drinks accounts for just over 2 per cent of total UK industrial activity.
–In 1980, total exports of alcoholic drinks amounted to £880 million.
–In 1980–81, the excise duties and VAT on alcoholic drinks are estimated to have raised £4000 million (i.e. 6 per cent of Central Government revenue).

The Government

Poised between the alcohol industry and the public health lobby is the Government: 18 different Government departments have some interest in alcohol.

Government departments concerned with alcohol

Department of Health and Social Security Trends in the effects of alcohol consumption. Health and social service provision for patients with alcohol problems. Health education on alcohol. Sponsoring research into alcohol abuse and related problems.

Ministry of Agriculture, Fisheries and Food Sponsorship of alcohol industry, including distribution and retailing. International aspects, trade, that bear on the well-being of industry. Regulation of drinks for purity, etc. Nutritional aspects of alcohol consumption.

Home Office Licensing laws. Offences of drunkenness. Other criminal offences associated with consumption of alcohol and treatment of offenders with alcohol problems. Police interest in drink-related road accidents. Broadcast advertising of alcoholic drinks.

Law Commission Office Functions of JPs in licensing laws.

Department Of Transport Road accidents and related legislation (Great Britain, in association with the Scottish Office).

Department of the Environment Football hooliganism, as affected by alcohol (with Home Office). Sponsorship of sport by alcohol industry.

Customs and Excise Duties on alcoholic drinks, including international negotiations.

Treasury Fiscal policy. Prices. Balance of payments for trade in alcohol. Economic significance of alcohol industry. Public expenditure effects of alcohol abuse.

Department of Trade Prices. Competition and pricing policy as it bears on the alcohol industry, including distribution and retailing. Policy on container sizes and metrication. Consumers' interest in advertising and promotion. International trade in alcoholic drinks. Press and cinema film industries. Alcohol consumption in the Merchant Navy and the civil aviation industry. Tourism.

Department of Employment Effect of alcohol abuse on accidents, absenteeism, and productivity.

Department of Education and Science Health education in schools. Effect on alcohol on young people in education.

Civil-Service Department Effect of alcohol abuse on the efficiency and conduct of the civil service.

Ministry of Defence Policies affecting the control of alcohol in the Armed Services and the treatment of its misuse.

Office of Population Censuses and Surveys Undertake studies on alcohol consumption and publish statistics on the harm due to alcohol.

Foreign Office Trade, international agreements.

Scottish Office

Welsh Office

Northern-Ireland Departments

In 1987, the Government initiated the Wakeham Committee to co-ordinate its response to alcohol problems.

The health lobby

The national public health lobby is small and poorly funded in comparison to the alcohol industry.

Action on Alcohol Abuse (AAA). 11 Carteret Street, London SW1H 9DL, is a campaigning organisation funded by the medical colleges to promote policies for reducing problems associated with alcohol consumption.

Alcohol Concern. 305 Gray's Inn Road, London WC1X 8QF was set up in 1984 and is funded by the Government to act as a forum for the dissemination of information about the harmful consequences of excessive drinking and to promote the development of preventive and therapeutic services for alcohol-related problems.

Alcohol Concern has a regional network based on regional health authorities.

References

Davies, P. and Walsh, D. (1983). Alcohol problems and alcohol control policies in Europe. Croom Helm, London.

Goddard, E. (1986). *Drinking and attitudes in licensing in Scotland.* Her Majesty's Stationery Office, London.

Thorley, A. (1985). The role of mass media campaigns in alcohol health education. In *The misuse of alcohol* (ed. N. Heather, I. Robertson, and P. Davies). Croom Helm, London.

Van Iwaarden, T. (1983). Advertising, alcohol consumption and policy alternatives. In *Economics and alcohol: Consumption and controls* (ed. M. Grant, M. Plant, and A. Williams). Croom Helm, London.

Appendix I: Further information

Books, reports, courses

British Medical Journal (1988). *Alcohol problems*. London, *BMJ*.
This book includes articles published in the *British Medical Journal*, practical articles written under the *ABC of Alcohol* series and an introductory article by Richard Smith on the public health aspects of alcohol.

Camberwell Council on Alcoholism (1980). *Women and alcohol*. London, Tavistock.
Women and alcohol is a collective book presenting current scientific research and thinking on a range of aspects on women's views of alcohol and its subsequent problems.

Edwards, G. (1987). *The treatment of drinking problems*. Grant MacIntyre, London.
This is the second edition of this book, which is a guide for the helping professions. It gives a clear background to the understanding of drinking problems, how to assess patients with drinking problems, and how to offer help to those at risk.

Grant, M. and Ritson, B. (1983). *Alcohol—the prevention debate*. Croom Helm, London.
This book presents different strategies for the prevention of alcohol-related harm and reviews their merits.

Heather, N. and Robertson, I. (1983). *Controlled drinking*. Methuen, London.

This book is the most comprehensive review of the literature dealing with the ability of patients with severe alcohol problems to achieve controlled drinking rather than abstinence.

Heather, N., Robertson, I., and Davies, P. (eds) (1985). *The misuse of alcohol.* Croom Helm, London.
This publication is a review of crucial issues related to dependence treatment and prevention of alcohol problems.

Orford, J. (1985). *Excessive appetites. A psychological view of Addictions.* John Wiley, Chichester.
This title develops a psychological understanding of a range of addictive behaviours or excessive appetites, including alcohol, drugs, food, gambling, and sexuality.

Orford, J. and Harwin, J. (eds) (1982). *Alcohol and the family.* Croom Helm, London.
This book is a collection of papers on the role that the family plays both in the origins of alcohol use and problem drinking, and in the ways in which the family can help individuals who are drinking excessively reduce their consumption.

Robinson, D. and Tether, P. (1986). *Preventing alcohol problems—A guide to local action.* Tavistock, London.
This is a very practical and comprehensive review of what can be done at a local level to prevent alcohol problems.

Royal College of General Practitioners. (1986). *Alcohol—A balanced review.* Report from General Practice, Royal College of General Practitioners, London.
This is a comprehensive practical guide to the prevention of alcohol problems in general practice listing what people drink; the reasons why people drink; the harms associated with alcohol; how to assess individual patients; how to give advice to those who are drinking excessively; how to prevent alcohol problems and examples of education, audit and research.

Royal College of Psychiatrists. (1986). *Alcohol—Our favourite drug.* Tavistock, London.
This is the second report on alcohol and alcohol-related problems from a special committee of the Royal College of Psychiatrists. It is a wide-ranging review of the problems that alcohol causes to society

and how they might be prevented.

Royal College of Physicians (1987). *The medical consequences of alcohol abuse—A great and growing evil.* Tavistock, London.
This book reviews, in an easy to understand manner, the medical harms related to alcohol consumption.

Sherlock, S. (ed.) (1982). *Alcohol and disease.* British Medical Bulletin, London.
This is a scientific review of a number of aspects of alcohol and disease.

Stockwell, T. and Clement, S. (eds) (1987). *Helping the problem drinker—New initiatives in community care.* Croom Helm, London.
This is a comprehensive up-to-date review of initiatives in community care for individuals with drinking problems. It discusses early interventions in general practice, the community and general hospitals, and considers the role of community agents and specialist community services in helping individuals with drinking problems.

World Health Organization (1985). *Alcohol policies. WHO regional publications,* European Series No. 18. WHO Regional Office for Europe, Geneva.
This is a comprehensive review of what can be done at a national level to prevent alcohol problems.

Drug use and misuse
This is a new course from The Open University in conjunction with the Health Education Authority. Its aim is to encourage improved practice in the field of alcohol and drugs by promoting greater understanding about the nature and role of drugs in society. The Individual Study Pack (price £35) includes a student study text booklet, an audio cassette, and a course reader. In addition, the group study pack (price £95) includes a video cassette and a group work booklet. The course, P576, is available from the Department of Health and Social Welfare, The Open University, Walton Hall, Milton Keynes MK7 6AA. Tel: 0908–653743.

Journals

The British Medical Journal frequently publishes articles related to alcohol and alcohol problems. In addition there are two specialist journals in the UK related to alcohol problems. The first is *The British Journal of Addiction*, published monthly, and is sent free to members of the Society for the Study of Addiction to Alcohol and Other Drugs. Requests for membership to the Society should be sent to:

Society for the Study of Addiction
c/o Carfax Publishing Company
P.O. Box 25, Abingdon
Oxfordshire OX14 3UE
(Subscription charge: £25 per year)

The second journal is *Alcohol and Alcoholism*—the International Journal of the Medical Council on Alcoholism. It is published bi-monthly and is sent to members of the Medical Council on Alcoholism, at a subscription charge of £20 per year.

Other addresses

Alcohol Concern
305 Gray's Inn Road
London WC1X 8QF
Tel: 01–833–3471

Alcohol Concern is the national agency on alcohol use and its problems. Alcohol Concern has an interest in the prevention of alcohol problems and the provision of services.

Action on Alcohol Abuse (AAA)
11 Carteret Street
London SW1H 9DL
Tel: 01–222–3454

AAA is a lobbying organization whose aim is to promote a healthy life-style by increasing public knowledge of the dangers of excessive drinking and to halt the current growth in consumption through equitable and effective control policies.

Medical Council on Alcoholism
1 St. Andrews Place
London NW1 4LP
Tel: 01–487–4445

The Medical Council on Alcoholism is the medical body which has a responsibility to ensure the undergraduate and postgraduate education and training of the medical profession about alcohol problems. The Council has produced a handbook for general practitioners called *Hazardous drinking.*

Appendix II: Reading for patients

The following are self-helps book for individuals to cut down on their drinking.

Chick, J. and Chick, J. (1984). *Drinking problems. Patient handbook 19.* Churchill Livingstone, Edinburgh.

Drink watchers' handbook (1985). A guide to healthy enjoyment of alcohol and how to achieve sensible drinking skills. Available from: ACCEPT Services, 2000 Seagrave Road, London SW6 1RQ.

Eastman, C. (1984). *Drink and drinking problems.* Longman, London.

Grant, M. (1984). *A guide to safer drinking.* Penguin, Harmondsworth.

Miller, W. and Munoz, R. (1982). *How to control your drinking.* Sheldon Press, London.

Robertson, I. and Heather, N. (1984). *So you want to cut down your drinking—A self-help guide to sensible drinking.* The Scottish Health Education Group, available from: The Scottish Health Education Group, Woodburn House, Canaan Lane, Edinburgh EH10 4SG.

Robertson, I. and Heather, N. (1986). *Let's drink to your health—A self-help guide to sensible drinking.* The British Psychological Society, available from: Distribution Centre, Black Horse Road, Letchworth, Hertfordshire SG6 1HN. Price: £3.95.

The following books are useful background reading for both patients and their carers:

Heather, N. and Robertson, I. (1985). *Problem drinking—The new approach.* Penguin, Harmondsworth.

Plant, M.A. (ed.) (1982). *Drinking and problem drinking.* Junction Books, London.

Plant, M.A. (1987). *Drugs in perspective.* Hodder and Stroughton, London.

Index

abstinence 57
accidents 27
action 56
Action on Alcohol Abuse 80, 85
advertising 72, 77
Alcohol Concern 80, 84
alcohol
  measurement card 36
  meters 39
  treatment units 63
Alcoholics Anonymous 63

blood
  pressure 25, 30
  tests 41–2, 54, 56, 60

CAGE 38
cancer 26
children 20
cirrhosis 3, 4, 12, 13, 14, 25, 29
community alcohol teams 63
consumer expenditure 7
consumption 6, 8–10
coronary heart disease 32–3
costs 1
councils on alcohol 62
crime 20
Cut Down on Your Drinking 50–1

DRAMS scheme 66
denial 34
diazepam 64–6
drink diary 46, 48, 54, 56, 58, 60
drinks trade 78
driving 21
drugs 23, 28
drunkeness 21

European Community 75
excise 78

family 17, 61
frequency/quantity question 36

gamma-gt 42, 54, 60, 69
government 78–9

Health Education Authority 44
health education 77
health service 1
hospitals 1, 68

income 6

licensing 73, 75–6

MAST 38
MCV 41–2, 54
MRC 67
Malmo 69
media 72
Medical Council on Alcoholism 85
memory 23
mortality 1, 4, 30, 31

occupation 13, 16

patient participation 73
peer group 12
pre-understanding 56
pregnancy 27, 30
price 6, 74–5
questionnaires 35, 36, 38–9

records 52
regional 10
relapse 61
risk 29

screening instrument 38
sexual function 26–7
smoking 66
social class 10
strokes 25
suicides 22

That's The Limit 44, 51

understanding 56
unemployment 10
units of alcohol 30, 49, 51

vitamins 65

women 9, 13, 30
World Health Organisation 38